breathe your way through birth with yoga

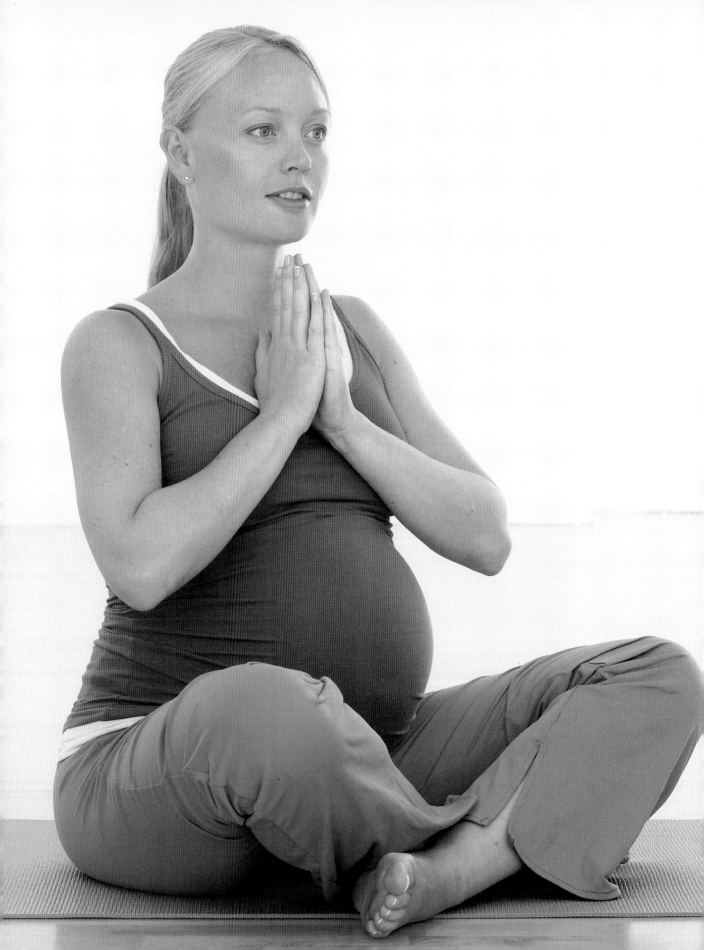

breathe your way through birth with yoga

Julie Llewellyn-Thomas

photography by Ruth Jenkinson

MITCHELL BEAZLEY

For my children – Clara, Rafi, Gabriel, and Lucia

First published in Great Britain in 2007 by Mitchell Beazley
An imprint of Octopus Publishing Group Ltd,
2–4 Heron Quays, Docklands, London E14 4JP

The views and advice expressed in this book are those of the author and based on her expertise as a practising yoga teacher and mother, having worked with many women and their partners during and after pregnancy with the yoga techniques described. While the advice and information in this book is believed to be accurate at the time of going to press, no legal responsibility or liability can be accepted by the publisher for any errors or omissions that may be made. This book is not intended as a substitute for professional medical advice where necessary and appropriate. As with any exercise programme it is advisable for the reader to consult with their medical practitioner and/or health visitor in all matters relating to the health of themselves and their baby and particularly in respect of any symptoms which may require diagnosis or medical attention prior to embarking on any exercise programme.

ISBN 13: 978 1 84533 272 3
ISBN 10: 1 84533 272 5

A CIP record for this book is
available from the British Library

Commissioning Editor Jonathan Asbury
Art Director Tim Foster
Designer Nicky Collings
Production Faizah Malik
Photographer Ruth Jenkinson
Senior Editor Hannah McEwen
Copy Editor Theresa Bebbington
Proofreader Alyson Lacewing
Index Ann Parry

Typeset in Perpetua
Produced by Toppan Printing Co., (HK) Ltd
Printed and bound in China

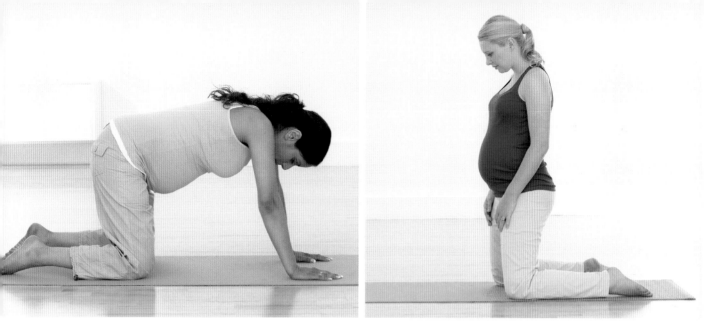

Contents

Birthing traditions

The way in which women give birth varies according to the culture and society in which they live. This is true both today and in the past. Thinking about how our mothers and grandmothers gave birth, we can picture our places in the current of history and realize how the distinct practices of our times affect us. These practices have influenced the choices that we can make when giving birth to our babies.

In some traditional societies, a woman prepares for birth by allowing her body to open up, ready for the release of the child. She symbolically clears the way, avoiding any thoughts or actions that may lead to obstruction or closure. The woman often gives birth in her own home, with a midwife and several elders. She is the centre, and the process revolves around her own pace. In contrast to the limiting "flat on the back" position often adopted during birth in the modern Western world, as long ago as 5750 BC women in Turkey gave birth more freely in the squatting position. In ancient Egypt, women knelt over two birthing bricks or sat on a brick seat, while birthing stools were commonplace in Greece and Rome.

In the Western world, the birthing stool, or chair, was used by midwives until the mid-18th century. Birth was viewed as a natural event and was managed by midwives, chosen from among the most trusted women in the neighbourhood. A warm, dark atmosphere was created, intended to ward off chills and to protect from evil spirits. A seated birth posture was usual, although this varied regionally. Labour was supported by the midwife and female relatives, but husbands might help in an emergency. Slow labours were sped by herbs and emetics, and midwives had "methods of version" to turn a badly positioned baby, as well as specific prayers and charms. Midwives were often victims of witch-hunts in the 17th century, as the church and scientific practice could not comprehend their female intuitive knowledge. The ancient spirituality that had accompanied birth was largely lost from the Western world.

In early 17th-century France, the Chamberlain brothers introduced the use of forceps, and this practice brought about a culture of requiring women to lie flat in bed during delivery. This fashion spread from the well-to-do to most classes of society, and physicians gradually took over from midwives in the birth chamber. The upright birthing chair fell out of general use by the end of the 18th century.

In the 19th century, the use of pain relief became widespread. Delivery under anaesthesia forced the trend towards giving birth while lying flat with the knees bent. Birth began to be seen as a medical complication, not a natural process. Opioid drugs and sedatives were first used in Austria in 1902. Women often had little memory of their labour, and later in the 20th century, when intravenous barbiturates were given, women were almost unconscious.

A RETURN TO NATURAL CHILDBIRTH

Up until the 1920s birth usually took place at home, with a midwife or doctor in attendance. After this time the new medical methods of "painless" childbirth in hospital took over, with the mother kept in a sterile environment and separated from the rest of the family, and these methods became the norm by the 1950s. As control passed from mothers and midwives to obstetricians, medical interventions became more common during labour, not only in emergencies but also as a matter of routine. It was also common for mothers to be separated from their babies after birth, disturbing the natural bonding between them.

This was a far cry from the practice of traditional cultures, where the midwife also plays a spiritual role, filling the woman with spiritual strength. By contrast, Western hospital practice was undermining mothers' trust and confidence in their own bodies, while physicians focused on possible problems and risks and doing tests. Opposition to medical birthing methods led to the formation of the Natural Childbirth Movement in Western societies. The English doctor Grantley Dick-Read, who wrote *Birth without Fear* in 1933, was a passionate champion of natural birth methods. Dick-Read believed that "even more important than the removal of pain is the spiritual joy the mother experiences when she sees her baby into the world, a joy which transcends the moment of birth, and has a lasting influence on family unity". He noted that if a mother's fear and tension could be reduced during labour, then pain would lessen too.

In 1947 the Russian psychiatrist Velvovski described a method of using deep breathing and therapeutic massage during contractions, to reduce stress and relieve pain. This technique was modified by Dr Fernand Lamaze in Paris in the early 1950s. Lamaze introduced antenatal classes, breathing practice, and relaxation training, which included the birth partner.

Natural childbirth is not new, but a return to some of the traditional practices, including upright birthing. Remember, however, that nature isn't always kind during birth, and that medical intervention can reduce risks to you and your baby in certain circumstances.

Today, as a mother, you are empowered to give birth in your own way and have a greater range of choices than ever before to meet your individual birthing needs. Society, while retaining the benefits of modern medicine, is rediscovering the sense of enchantment that accompanies birthing, the sense of the elemental forces of creation and the warm touch of mother, baby, and partner. Yoga, a traditional practice that brings harmony between the mother, baby, and partner, is a natural birth companion.

BELOW Practising with your partner during pregnancy will help you feel less stressed, which can only be better for your baby.

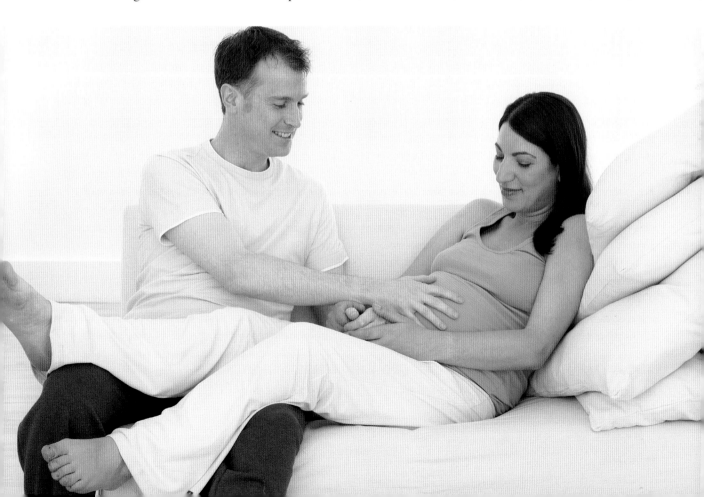

What is yoga?

The origins of yoga can be traced back to ancient Hindu India, where its traditions and practices have been handed on from person to person by word of mouth for more than 5,000 years. The word "yoga" is derived from *yug*, a Sanskrit word meaning "union". In yoga, the union is between body, mind, and spirit, as well as the dedication of the self to a way of life.

Yoga can have a strong spiritual element for those who explore its depths, based on the togetherness of all things – living and non-living – in the universe. Yoga is not a religion as such, but many people – both ancient and modern – have found fulfilment in its alertness and tranquillity, its physical activity, and the deep relaxation it brings.

Yoga encourages people of whatever conviction to believe in their own potential, to develop themselves through a combination of physical postures (*asanas*), breathing exercises (*pranayama*), inner awareness (*dharana*), and meditation (*dhyana*). These are important aspects of the eight "arms" of yoga, described by the Indian sage Patanjali in his yoga sutras, which were written down in about the 2nd century AD. There are important ethical principles to follow, known as *yamas* and *niyamas*, which are "commandments" and "observances", with the end goal being *Samadhi*, which is many things – a state of peace and oneness with the universe, a refining of the mind. Some people may wish to be "yogis" in this way, bringing yoga into all aspects of their lives.

In the modern Western world, yoga is more often thought of as a way to increase your physical fitness, which is fine as it can improve body tone, posture, and stamina. You can do yoga as much or as little as you like to suit your needs, and you don't even need to chant if you feel uncomfortable with it. But whatever yoga you manage to do will bring a rest from the hectic rush of modern life. Yoga is non-competitive – it is about achieving harmony and well-being. It will improve your suppleness and strength, relax your mind, and improve your respiration and circulation. These things will benefit both you and your baby during birth, and later on during parenting.

THE ASPECTS OF YOGA

The 6th-century Indian text the *Bhagavad Gita* includes a discussion between the god Krishna and the warrior Arjuna on the nature of yoga, including its many aspects. Some of these you may find to be helpful during birth and labour:

- Yoga is serenity
- Yoga is the destroyer of pain
- Yoga is self-control
- Yoga is the producer of the greatest happiness
- Yoga is equilibrium in success and failure

In yoga the term "practice" refers to the time that you devote to yoga, or its content, not the practising to get things just right! There are various types of yoga in use today, which are derived from classical yoga. The postures in this book are based on gentle Hatha yoga, which focuses on synchronizing movement and breath without using strenuous movements.

You will often find that the postures, or *asanas*, used in yoga are referred to by their Sanskrit names, which are colourful and describe their resemblance to the shapes of animals or other natural things. Examples are *Tadasana*, the "mountain pose", and *Svanasana*, the "dog pose". This book uses their common English names for simplicity.

The *asanas* are what most people picture when thinking of yoga. They come from the Sanskrit word *as*, which means "to stay". Generally, you should hold each of these postures for a short while, keeping steady and comfortable, or better still, moving with your breath. However, remember you should never be shaking or in pain.

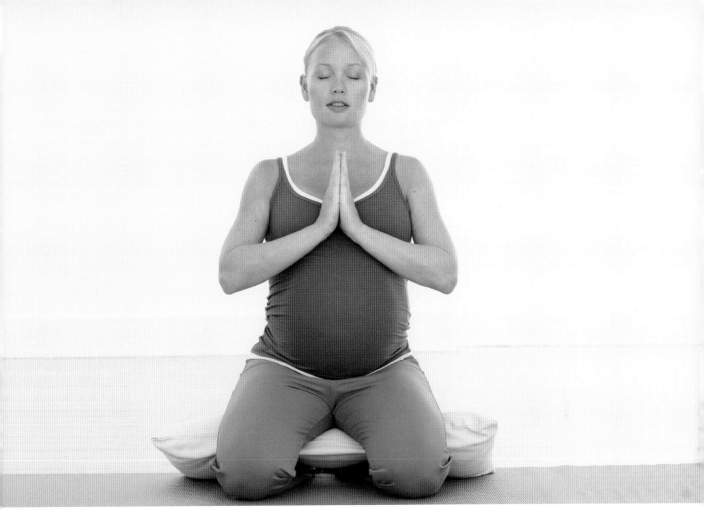

Breathing, or *pranayama*, is also fundamental to yoga. The term *prana* in Sanskrit refers to the "life force" or "energy", and *ayama* means a "release" or "stretching out". By using controlled breathing in yoga you are extending your life energy, as *prana* flows in to the body via the breath and is retained within you. You should be careful not to hold your breath or breathe in and out too rapidly. The aim is to achieve deep relaxation.

Breathing is normally focused on a gentle, slow in-breath and a long, slow out-breath, but in some practices may vary from a loud "ha!" to release tension, to sounds of humming bees or hissing snakes! The sound "ahh ... ohh ... mmm", which is used in this book, is based on that of the Sanskrit "aum" or "om", which is sacred in yoga and is a simple but universal mantra or chant, used to relax you, centre you, and turn you inwards to your deeper self.

There has been a large awakening of interest in yoga across the world in the last century, as it appeals to people from all backgrounds, living in many different situations, whatever their individual goals may be. Yoga is increasingly used for general health, for promoting fitness, mindfulness, and relaxation – and, of course, during pregnancy and giving birth.

TIP How you feel emotionally is very important, so don't practice if you feel angry or upset.

How yoga and breathing help you give birth

Yoga helps you stay fit and supple, it relaxes your body and mind, it gives you a break from the outside world, and it helps you become more aware of your body and your ability to control it. Although yoga wasn't designed to help with labour and childbirth – it was originally performed only by men – it might as well have been because each one of these benefits can make all the difference to a pregnant woman.

With yoga to help you, your birth can be a gentler and more beautiful experience – you will feel empowered to give birth in the way that's best for you, perhaps in an upright position. Evidence suggests that babies born in this way are healthier and more alert, and that mothers recover far more quickly. A positive birth experience will mean that you can give your baby the warmest of welcomes into the world and will strengthen the bonds between you.

Many yoga positions practised in pregnancy are similar to those that are helpful during labour and birthing. They can allow your pelvis to open up, help to position your baby properly, and prepare you psychologically to open and release while giving birth. Regular practise can help you to become familiar with positions such as squatting, kneeling, or on all fours, which will feel natural during labour and birth, because they allow gravity to assist your baby's passage. Indeed, many women have said that if they practise the gentle yoga positions during pregnancy, they have the confidence to move freely and spontaneously in labour. You do not need a special environment to practise yoga – you can kneel on a bed, support your hips against a wall, squat on the floor, or lie on your side. All this is comforting in labour – especially in an unfamiliar hospital room – and can help facilitate a birth. The benefits of yoga will also go beyond giving birth, and can stay with you for the rest of your life (see page 82).

THE BENEFITS OF YOGA
Yoga is the breath – the two cannot be separated. In yogic terms, you are measured not by how many years you live but by how many breaths you take. Longer and slower breaths will translate into a longer and calmer life. The breath offers a unique way to focus on turning inwards and is key to coping with labour pains. Deeper breathing with lengthened breaths will provide mental focus and increase endorphin levels, the natural "feel-good" pain inhibitors. And the more of those you can have during labour, the better!

Yoga offers different breathing practices, or *pranayama*, which are explained in this book. Most women will find these practices helpful during labour and birthing, as well as after the birth in order to stay relaxed when caring for a young baby. If you are angry or upset you will tighten your shoulders, grit your teeth, and breathe rapidly and shallowly. This in turn causes you to feel more anxious and increases tension in your body. By developing an awareness of your breath you can break the cycle, calming your body and mind (see pages 18–19).

YOGA AND GIVING BIRTH
During labour, especially if you are in hospital, in an unfamiliar environment surrounded by strangers, you will breathe more rapidly. If you are frightened or in pain, your breathing will be shallow. This quickened breathing can cause the stress hormone adrenaline to be produced and make contractions more painful.

By slowing down your breathing you are calming your emotions and having a positive physiological effect on your body. Relaxation and centring will subdue levels of adrenaline and promote the production of oxytocin, which is needed for effective contractions. This will enable you to work with your contractions rather than being overtaken by them. With yoga, you will be more serene during labour and birth, helping you to control your response to pain and relax between contractions, preserving your energy for when it is really needed.

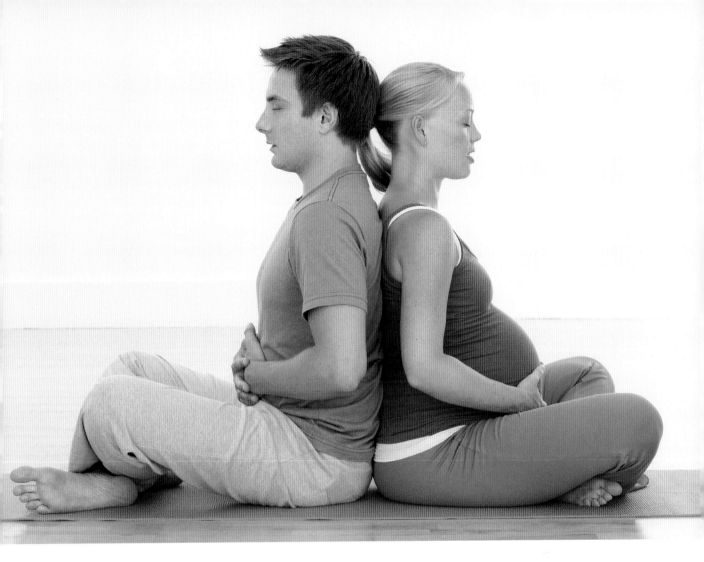

There is a link between relaxed mothers and relaxed babies, as the stress hormone cortisol may be passed between you. The breathing, stretching, and relaxation of yoga have a soothing effect on the body and the mind. Yoga is also an ideal way to develop healthier patterns of thought and behaviour and it develops self-awareness. By taking time out to focus on your breath, you will have a chance to turn inwards at a deep level, becoming more aware, physically and possibly spiritually. Whether you are excited or scared (or both!) about giving birth, yoga will support you during the transition to motherhood.

An important role of yoga is to keep the birth as relaxed as possible. If you have your baby in a hospital, yoga can support you throughout your labour as it can be used in any position, even if medical intervention is needed. You can carry yoga within you during the whole birth process to deepen your own inner strength. Even if there is trauma or the birth doesn't go to plan, whether at home or in hospital, you can use yoga to help you let go of disappointment and progress positively. Women who experience birth traumas may feel that they have not had the opportunity they would like to bond with their baby, and yoga can play an important part in this. Most importantly, enjoy yoga and the closeness it will bring between you, your partner, and your baby. This provides the best possible foundation for happy, healthy birthing and parenting.

The importance of the birth partner

The birth partner will physically and emotionally support the expectant mother. It's the partner's job to provide security and comfort during the birth. For the mother, having a supportive birth partner enables her to feel more in control of the process. The more empowered she feels during the birth, the better she will bond with the baby and the less likely she will feel depression afterwards.

Giving birth with yoga is for everyone, and this includes the birth partner. A partner who has been practising yoga with the expectant mother will be able to support her with more confidence during labour. Most women will choose someone close to them to accompany them through the journey of birth. For some this will be a female relation or possibly a best friend; however, many women will opt to be with their sexual partner. Whoever your partner is, his or her support can provide strength and confidence throughout the pregnancy and during the critical stages of labour.

The presence of a birth partner brings lots of benefits. These include psychological support for the mother and better communication with hospital staff. The birth partner will understand the mother's needs and know when to help – or even when to take a step back and let her have some time to herself. He or she can be the mother's advocate when speaking to health professionals, expressing what she may not be able to voice herself. He or she can prepare the mother for labour, as well as support her during the birth. The partner's presence also provides feelings of privacy and security. This in turn stimulates oxytocin release, which can help to create an easier birth. Research suggests that the presence of a birth partner is associated with less pain, panic, and exhaustion. Fewer epidurals are needed and labours are often shorter. It can also lower the rate of Caesarean sections and assisted deliveries.

As a birth partner you receive benefits too, such as the satisfaction of giving support, as well as being part of a "rite of passage" that sees the birth of a new life. No one would claim that the birth partner's role is easy. It's not just about learning techniques and breathing exercises – it's about knowing your partner's non-verbal behaviour, her wants, and her needs. It is not about being a "coach" – rather it enables her to find an active birth rhythm, with your support and reassurance. The shared practice of yoga will help you to know each other at a profound and deep level. As a birth partner, your love and support will help to create the right birthing environment, especially in a hospital. You can touch, massage, and hold the mother. But be flexible – no matter how long you have practised together prior to the birth, events may still surprise you. Go with the flow in response to her needs.

Not all women, however, wish to have their partner present at the birth. The mother has the right to choose what is best for her. Some health workers may even feel that a father's presence may be a hindrance if there are tensions in the relationship or he is squeamish when things are difficult.

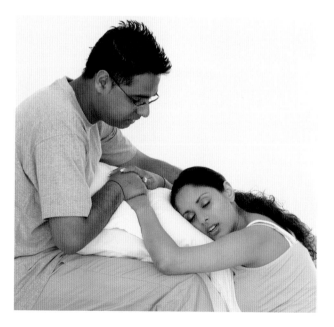

How to use this book

This book will guide you through breathing exercises and birthing positions derived from yoga postures to help and support you during labour and birth. Before you begin any of the practices make sure you have read the important guidelines on when to practise and when not to practise (see page 14). Then look at *Helpful hints for your birth* (see page 15), which will guide you through useful practicalities on how to make the best of your labour and birth – whether it's at hospital or at home.

- Using yoga exercises and breathing exercises, you will create your own sequences, which you should practise every day.

- The diagram below shows you how you can put a sequence together.

- By practising your sequence every day, you will be prepared for birth by being comfortable and ready for the positions and movements during each stage of labour. You will be able to choose your own labour and birth positions to suit you, drawing on the yoga and breathing you have learned.

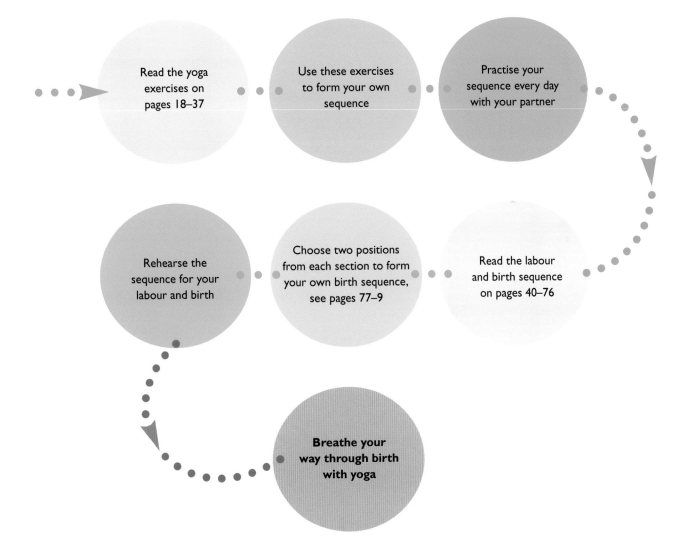

Read the yoga exercises on pages 18–37

Use these exercises to form your own sequence

Practise your sequence every day with your partner

Read the labour and birth sequence on pages 40–76

Choose two positions from each section to form your own birth sequence, see pages 77–9

Rehearse the sequence for your labour and birth

Breathe your way through birth with yoga

When to practise and when not to practise

Yoga can provide support and reassurance during your labour and the birth of your baby. You, your partner, and your baby will benefit so long as you follow these guidelines.

DO

- Practise your breathing. If you do nothing else, it's the breath that counts.

- Always take time to practise your yoga stretches and breathing exercises for 10 minutes at the same time each day, preferably with your partner. The more you practise breathing together, the easier it will be to use the yoga breath during your labour.

- Enjoy! Practise the sequences and enjoy the cuddles, the intimacy of the breathing, and the time together. The more joy you can get from your practice, the more likely you will be to use it during birthing.

- Always listen to your body. If you are trying out a yoga stretch, a birthing position, or a breathing exercise, and it doesn't feel comfortable – stop.

- Include siblings. Many brothers and sisters enjoy the yoga practice and it may help them understand the birth process and feel more confident about it.

- Make sure the room in which you are practising your yoga is warm, calm, and well ventilated.

- Always take off your shoes and socks and use a non-slip yoga mat for your yoga practice.

- Make sure you have all the equipment you need before you begin practising. You will need a chair, bean bag, bed, yoga mat, stool, and lots of cushions. Get familiar with these beforehand and you will feel comfortable with them during labour.

- Always check with your doctor or midwife if you feel unsure whether you should be doing any of the practices in this book.

DON'T

- Don't do anything that feels uncomfortable for you. This includes yoga stretches, breathing practices, and rehearsals for labour and birth.

- Never have a full stomach when practising yoga stretches, breathing practices, and rehearsals for labour and birth. You can eat a light snack beforehand, but you shouldn't have anything heavy.

- Never rush. If you are in a hurry leave your yoga practice for later.

- Don't worry if you haven't got time to try out every single labour or birthing exercise. Even if you focus on only one or two movements with your breathing practice, it will make a difference.

- Don't get too fixed in your ideas and expectations. Birth is unpredictable – you can make plans but sometimes things don't work out as you expect. Use your breathing practice to help relax you whatever the circumstances.

- Don't begin your yoga and breathing practices until you have taken a few moments to read about the benefits of yoga and breathing. The more you understand the benefits, the more you will be committed to practise.

Helpful hints for the birth

Giving birth is a highly instinctive process. You need to be allowed to turn deep inside yourself, looking to your yoga and breathing to support you through this journey. The following practicalities may be helpful in creating a secure, comfortable, private space for you to give birth. The more relaxed labour you have, the quicker it will proceed.

Whether you are having your baby at a hospital or in your home, it is important that you create a safe and secure atmosphere in which you will feel comfortable. Although this can be more difficult in hospital, you can bring along some home comforts such as a bean bag, cushions, your yoga mat, a CD player, or anything else that is important to you.

- Dim the lights if you are giving birth at home – candles can create a relaxed atmosphere. You won't be able to use candles in a hospital but you can try to turn off the lights. If this isn't possible and you need darkness, put a blanket or sheet over your head to shut out the outside world.
- Use a plug-in vaporizer with lavender oil to calm the atmosphere.

- Put your yoga mat and bean bag on the floor and scatter around some cushions. Make sure there is a chair in the room. If you have a low stool, you can supply that too, even if you are in hospital.
- If you are in hospital, lower the bed and put something on it so that you won't be tempted to use the bed unless you have to.
- Get rid of any white sheets or anything that makes you feel uncomfortable.
- Check that you have all your drinks and energizing snacks at hand.
- Make sure that any chatter and unnecessary conversation goes on outside the room, not in it. You need space to focus, and agitations, lack of privacy, and discomforts will only slow you down.

Waters, you are the ones who bring us the life force. Help us to find nourishment so that we may look upon great joy. *Rig Veda, Chapter 10, Hymn 9*

Preparing yourself

Preparing your mind and body

By practising yoga – either alone or with your partner – during the early stages of pregnancy, you are providing the best for your pregnancy and preparing yourself for giving birth and mothering. During your pregnancy you will find that yoga practice offers you "time out" to focus – you will learn to quietly turn inward, be more in tune with your body, focus on your breath, and be aware of your baby.

To use yoga positions and breathing effectively during your labour and birth, you need to do some preparation in pregnancy by doing a little gentle yoga practice every day. This yoga practice should include breathing exercises for centring, which will help you to calm down and focus on your physical postures (or *asanas*). You should also do a few warm-ups to release tension from your shoulders and jaw (see page 21). All these are essential during labour, as between contractions you will be tense – but the more relaxed you are, the easier and less painful labour will be.

Exercises that focus on the pelvis increase mobility in the joints, help your pelvis to "open up", and enhance circulation. When you practise the **tailor pose** (see page 22), **stirring the soup** (see page 22), and the **half lotus with flowing arms** (see page 23) you will notice improved flexibility, which is essential in pregnancy, during labour and birth.

Practise the postures that are similar to birth positions, some of which combine yoga stretches. The **rolling cat** (see page 24) is done on your hands and knees, and with practise it can become instinctive during labour, perhaps on your yoga mat or on the bed. It focuses on movement in the spine, combining your movement with your breath. You will find that your breath automatically begins to lengthen. You can use this practice during labour and giving birth.

BELOW By practising yoga together you are preparing not only for the challenges of labour, but for the new role of parenting that lies ahead of you.

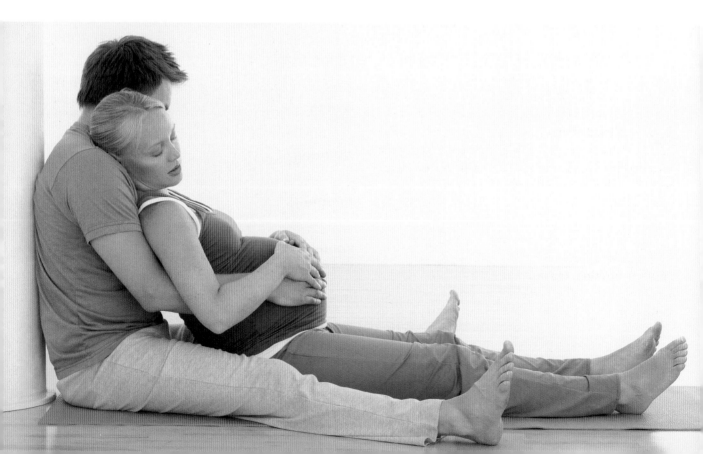

Being on your hands and knees and then **resting forward on a bean bag** (see page 47) is perfect for labour. It encourages your baby to lie in the best possible position ready for birth (the *occipito-anterior* position – with your baby's back facing toward your front). Any leaning forward posture will encourage your baby to lie in this position. This is important, as the alternative position (the *occipito-posterior* position – with your baby's back against your spine) can result in a longer, slower, and more "back-achey" type of labour.

OTHER POSES

The **supported hero's pose** (see page 25) is a comfortable position with supported feet. If you familiarize yourself with this position, you will feel comfortable either going into a **mini squat** (see page 26), which is ideal for birthing, or you can lean forward onto bean bags and focus on contractions. **Kneeling with circling hips** (see page 26), as well as **half kneeling and half squatting** (see page 29), are essential to practise for labour and birth if you feel comfortable on your knees. These positions are comfortable when supported and yet provide optimum space, and make use of gravity for a birth.

The **mountain pose** (see page 27) focuses on good posture. The better your posture during pregnancy, the less likely you are to experience aches and pains in your pelvis and lower back. By learning to stand tall and erect you are distributing your weight equally and will carry your baby with ease. Your more open posture, free from hunching, will improve your breathing. Unrestricted breathing is important, as your baby will benefit from the richer oxygen supply.

The **moving squats** (see page 27) are a gentle way to include movement while you practise the squatting position. You can use squatting in labour and birthing, and you may find that you suddenly find comfort in a squat while walking around the room.

If your partner needs a stretch too, try the **back stretch with partners** (see page 28), where you stretch forward and extend your lower back and shoulders, while your partner enjoys a mini squat. Your partner can also do the back stretch against a wall on his own if he is tired and needing revitalizing.

Don't forget to practise your pelvic floor exercises every day – these are done in the knee to chest position (see page 30), helping you focus on your pelvic floor and can also be useful if your labour is coming fast and you want to slow it down. The more you know your pelvic floor, the easier it will be for you to release the muscles to help you birth more gently.

Choose a breathing exercise (see pages 32–37). You need to choose only one or two. It may be a breathing exercise to do alone or with your partner. You will learn to let go of any tensions and focus on your breath, an essential skill for labour and birthing.

SAFETY TIPS FOR STRETCHING OUT

- Focus on long, slow breaths. Unlike traditional yoga, breathe in through your nose and breathe out from your mouth to prepare for labour.

- Don't hold a pose for too long. Let your breathing be your guide. The key is to breathe freely – if your breathing is restricted, you should come out of the position immediately.

- Focus on the natural curves of your spine. Imagine you have a large tail that is tucking under and drawing your bottom to the ground.

- Spread out your hands and fingers when you are on your hands and knees – this will protect your wrists from injury.

- Don't hurry your practice. Unplug the phone and tell everyone that you want to be left undisturbed.

Centring ▶

Try to centre yourself at the start of a session, using the following routine:

1 Sit comfortably and upright, focusing your mind on your breathing.

2 Put your hands on your rib cage and gently follow your breathing, being aware of its rise and fall. Don't hurry: allow each breath to be fully exhaled before you inhale again.

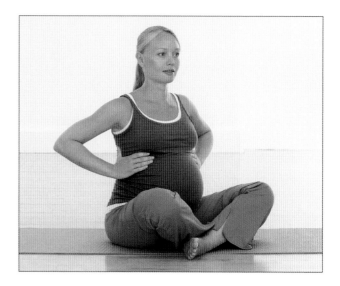

Breathing arms ▼

In this flowing movement, work on expanding your out breath. By breathing in deeply, stretching up to the sky, and opening your chest, you are filling yourself and your baby with *prana* (universal energy). By releasing a big out-breath from your mouth, you are releasing any tension and will begin to relax, eventually finding inner harmony.

1 Sit on the floor with your back upright and your legs either crossed or straight out in front of you. Bring your palms together in a prayer pose. Take a moment to get comfortable – you can do this with your partner's back against yours.

2 When you're ready, with the next in breath, take your arms up above your head.

3 As you release your arms to your sides let out a loud out breath. Bring your palms back into the prayer pose. Repeat 4 to 6 times, each time deepening your in breath and extending your out breath.

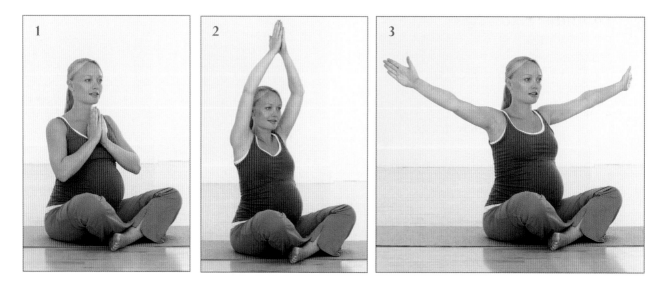

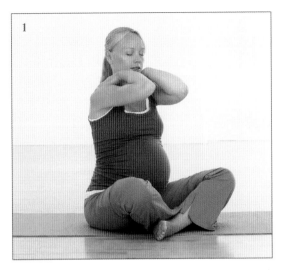

◄ Shoulder openers

1 Remain sitting in a comfortable position. Place your fingertips on your shoulders.

2 Make large, slow circles with your elbows so that your shoulders rotate fully in their sockets. As you breathe in, take your elbows up to the ceiling and as you breathe out, take them back down. Repeat this a few times forward and then do it backward. You should feel warmer across the front of your chest and across your upper back.

TIP Not everyone feels comfortable sitting upright on a yoga mat. If you find it difficult to keep your back straight, try sitting on the very edge of a cushion or pillow.

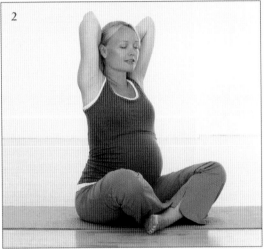

Shoulder releases ►

1 Sit comfortably and upright, breathe in and draw your shoulders up to your ears.

2 As you breathe out, allow your shoulders to drop and let out your breath with a loud "ha!" sound.

TIP Make sure you are wearing comfortable clothing that won't restrict your movements.

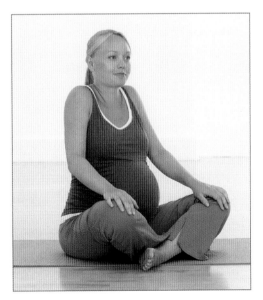

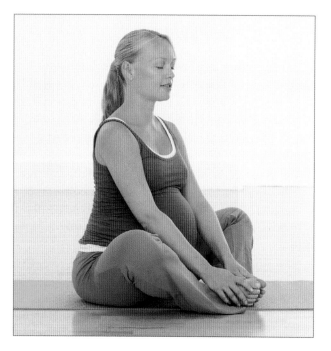

◄ Tailor pose

The tailor pose will open your whole pelvic region, your inner thighs, and your hips. It is used to encourage good reproductive health in both women and men, and is beneficial during pregnancy and birth.

1 Sit comfortably and upright. Gently bring the soles of your feet together and hold them lightly with your hands.

2 Breathe in deeply. As you breathe out, allow your knees to rest gently toward the ground, but don't force them down or strain them.

TIP For extra support when doing the tailor pose, try it with your back against the wall or place cushions under your knees.

Stirring the soup ►

This invigorating pose stretches out and strengthens the upper body while bringing mobility and flexibility to the lower body. Be careful not to overstretch.

1 Sit comfortably and upright with your legs apart. For extra comfort place a small cushion under your buttocks. Stretch your arms out and place your hands together as if you were holding a big soup spoon. Turn your toes gently upward.

2 Breathe in deeply and stretch your hands toward your right foot. Breathe out and draw your hands to your left foot, then to your waist, and back to your right foot.

3 Repeat a few times, and then reverse the direction, breathing long, slow breaths.

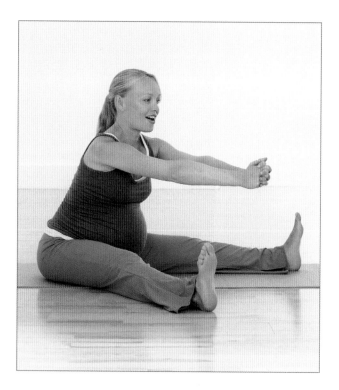

Half lotus with flowing arms ▼

This elegant pose stretches the inner thigh, expands the chest, and improves your breathing.

1 Sit comfortably and upright with your legs apart. Move your right foot close to your left inner thigh (you can place a supportive cushion under your knee). Sit tall and breathe a few long, slow breaths.

2 Slowly reach forward with your left arm and hold on to your left leg to stretch your hamstring. Allow your head to relax forward and breathe slowly.

3 As you breathe in, reach your right arm toward your left foot, then raise it up. As you release a big out breath take your arm up and behind you.

4 Breathing in, sweep your arm forward toward your left leg, and breathe out. Repeat several times, before resting forward and allowing your breath to return to normal. Repeat on the other side.

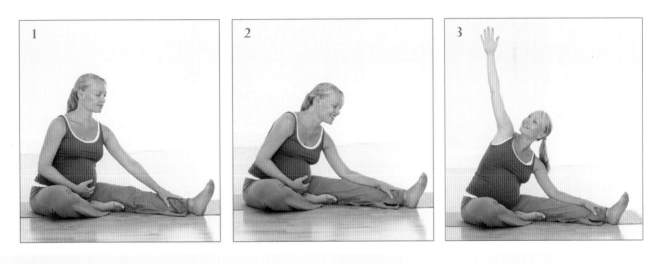

Rolling cat ▼

The rolling cat should consist of continuous flowing movements.

1 Start on all fours on a mat, breathing normally.

2 As you breathe out, tuck your bottom under, round your back, tuck your chin in and drop your bottom to your heels. Allow your breath to release fully.

3 Breathing in, drop your elbows to the ground, before rounding your back once more to return

to the start position (see photo 1). Continue this slow flowing movement as many times as you feel comfortable with, keeping the movement in time with your breath.

4 Finally, take a few moments to rest with your head relaxed and your arms stretched out in front of you (in a supported child pose). You can try using a bean bag if you need some extra support, making sure your feet are comfortable and you have enough support for your head.

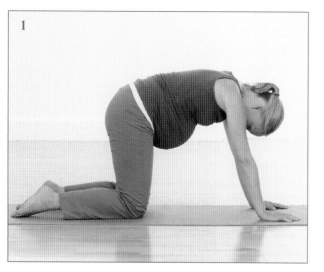

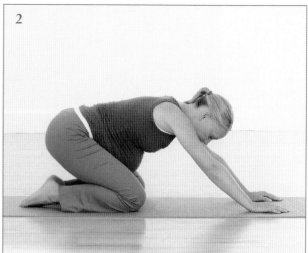

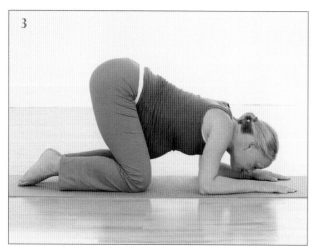

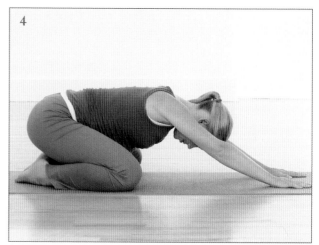

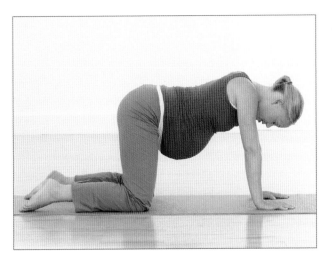

◄ Moving hips with sound

1 Start on all fours, with your knees under your hips and hands spread wide as if you have tiger paws.

2 Gently move your hips in a circle. Allow your jaw to be loose, your face relaxed, and your neck soft. Slowly breathe a deep in breath and as you breathe out release a big "ahhh" or another sound. Repeat a few times and don't rush. Rest in the supported child pose as in step 4 of the **rolling cat** (see opposite page).

Supported hero's pose ►

The hero's pose is comfortable for resting and quietening the mind, and can be used during labour by leaning forward on a bean bag or a chair (see page 47). Place a cushion between your bottom and your heels, and under your feet too if it feels comfortable.

1 Sit in a kneeling position with your knees slightly apart and your bottom touching your heels. Your buttocks should rest on your feet or a cushion. Make sure your back is relaxed and your spine is as straight as possible.

2 Bring your palms together in the prayer position and breathe long slow breaths toward your palms. With each out breath, press your palms together, and feel the strength of your exhalation.

TIP If you have varicose veins, avoid staying in this position for long periods of time.

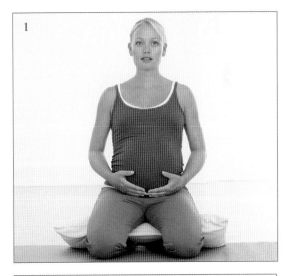

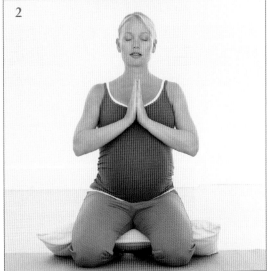

Mini squats from hero pose ▾

This is a gentle supported squat that you can use in labour. It focuses on making space for your baby and encourages the baby to be in the best position before the birth.

1 Sit in the **supported hero's pose** (see page 25). Raise your left leg to bend it into a mini squat, keeping your left knee in line with your left ankle.

2 Lower your right buttock toward your right heel, and lean forward onto your hands. Your buttocks may lift up but this is fine. Gently move your body in little circles, focusing on long, slow breaths.

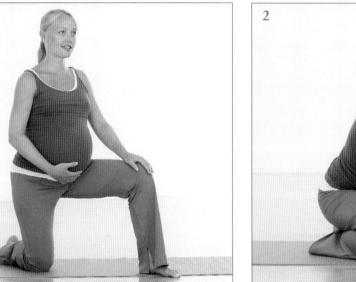

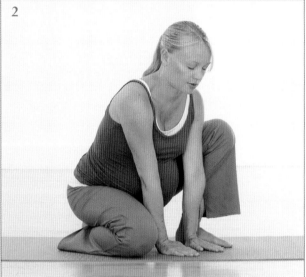

Kneeling with circling hips ▸

Many women find this position helpful during labour and for birthing itself. If you have a knee injury or have had a knee operation, don't attempt it.

1 Go up onto your knees, allowing them to be slightly apart.

2 Bring your hands to your baby and gently move your hips in a circular motion. Focus on your breath. You can breathe a deep in breath and long, slow out breath, or focus on your sound breath.

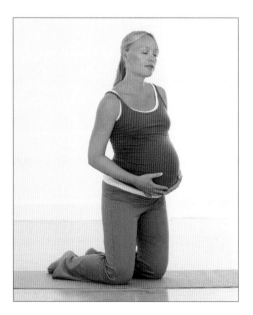

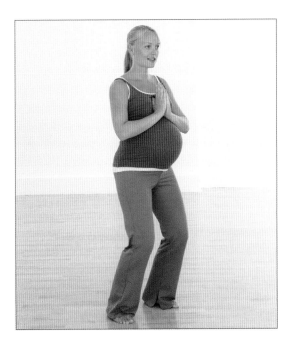

◄ Mountain pose

The mountain pose forms the foundation of all standing poses in pregnancy. The key is to support your posture and make space for your baby.

1 Stand upright with your feet positioned under your hips and your knees slightly bent. Place your hands in the prayer position. Make sure that your jaw is relaxed, that your chest is open by pulling your shoulders back, and that you are standing upright.

2 Breathe long, slow breaths, allowing yourself to grow tall with each in breath and feel firmly grounded with each out breath.

Moving squats ▼

1 Stand in the **mountain pose**, and bring your hands into the prayer position (see above). As you breathe in raise your arms above your head.

2 As you breathe out bring your arms down and out to the side, and bend your knees into a gentle squat.

3 Slowly bring your palms back into the prayer position. Repeat this a few times if you feel comfortable. Avoid going too fast and enjoy the flowing movement.

TIP Don't practise squats if you have any pain in your groin or hips. You don't have to squat deeply.

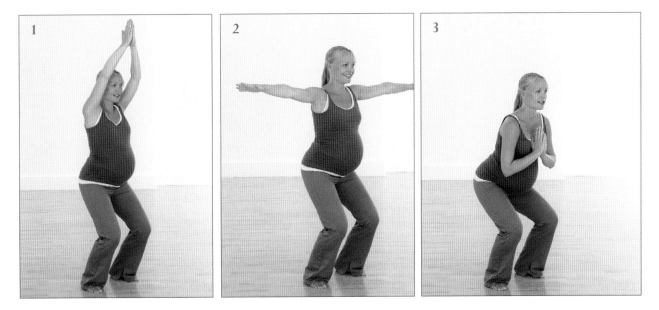

Back stretch with partner ▼

This is a wonderful opportunity to stretch with your partner. This sequence combines a supported squat with a back stretch. Both exercises stretch the body and improve stamina. Remember to come out of the pose gently and don't suddenly let go of your partner when you've had enough!

1 Face your partner and hold on to each others' arms.

2 Ask your partner to slowly bend his knees and go into a gentle supported squat, while you walk your legs back until your back is flat like a table top, keeping your knees a little bent.

3 Try adjusting yourselves – ask your squatting partner to relax his shoulders and loosen his jaw, and make sure he is sitting back as if he is avoiding sitting on a toilet seat. Now ask your partner to pull your arms until you feel a gentle stretch in your upper back and shoulders. Keep your arms aligned straight and your head relaxed. Talk to each other to make sure you are both okay. Breathe a couple of long, slow breaths.

4 When you are both ready, slowly walk your legs in while your partner comes out of the squat gently. Give your bodies a little shake, relaxing your shoulders, arms, and legs. Then change over and swap your positions.

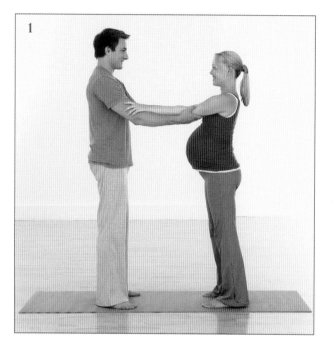

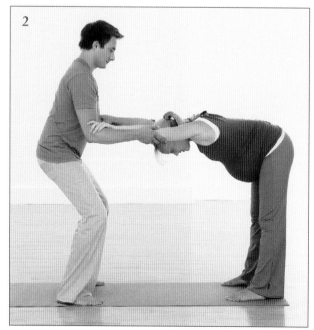

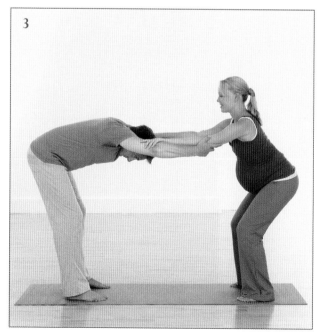

Half kneeling and half squatting ▶

This is a lovely pose that can be done during labour on the floor, on your yoga mat. You can lean forward onto a bed or bean bag in this pose (see page 65). You can also use it for birthing as it provides lots of space for your baby and makes good use of gravity.

1 Sit in the **supported hero's pose** (see page 25). Gently come up into a kneeling position, and raise your left leg to bend it into a mini squat, keeping your left knee in line with your left ankle. Use a chair or wall for support if you need to.

2 Placing your left hand on your left knee, gently lean forward and move your hips in a circular motion. Be aware of your breath and rest your hands on your baby if you want.

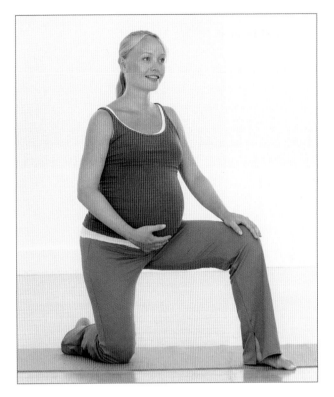

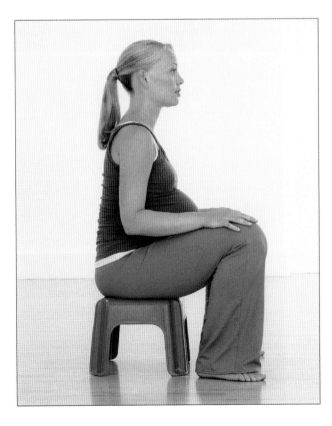

◀ Mini squats on a stool

1 Place a low stool behind you, making sure that it is stable

2 Stand with your feet a little apart, in line with your hips. Gently drop your weight into your heels and then – keeping your heels flat on the floor – bend your knees, lengthen your lower back. and lower yourself slowly into a squat with your buttocks resting on the stool. Turn your feet and knees out if you want.

3 Stay here for as long as it feels comfortable, then come up slowly and gently.

TIP Don't practise these squats if you have any pain in your groin or hips.

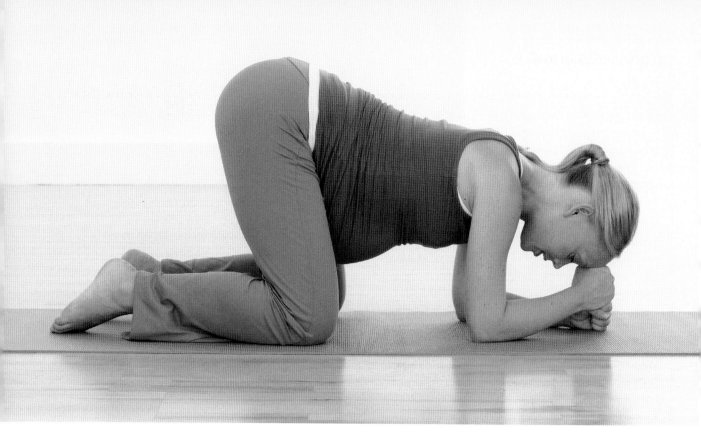

Pelvic floor exercises ▲

With good preparation in pregnancy and sensible use of upright positions during the birth, the pelvic floor – the muscles in the pelvic area – should stay strong and healthy. Regular pelvic floor exercises during pregnancy will allow you to become aware of your pelvic floor, learning to release its muscles, which is essential for birthing.

1 Practise the exercises in the knee to chest position, as shown above. In this position your chest will lower, and be closer to the ground. You can use this position during labour should it be going too fast and you need to slow things down (see page 58).

2 Focus on the area around your anus. Breathe in and draw it in, breathe out and release. Repeat this a few times.

3 Move to your urethra. If you focus on your clitoral area, this can help guide you to the right place. Do some quick movements, squeezing and releasing repeatedly. Repeat this a few times. If you have trouble locating the area imagine that you are stopping your flow of urine mid-stream when you are on the toilet.

4 Now focus on your vagina. Breathe in and gently draw the area in, breathe out and release. Repeat this a few times.

5 Finally, focus on your whole pelvic floor – the three areas all together. Breathe in, draw the areas in, breathe out and gently release.

Joined relaxation ▾

This simple five-minute routine is an ideal way for you and your partner to share relaxation together. Joined relaxation is worth learning for future days together, especially as parents. If you want, you can tape these instructions to listen to until you can remember them.

1 Lie on your left-hand side with your partner lying behind you. Your partner can either wrap his arms around you with his hands on your baby or you may prefer just to hold hands. Make sure you are both comfortable. Put a cushion between your knees and under your heads if you need to. You could even cover yourselves with a blanket. Turn off the phone.

2 Begin your relaxation by breathing a deep in breath. When you breathe out release a big "ha!" breath. Repeat a few times, trying to release any tension.

3 Begin to follow your breath, both your in breath and your out breath. Try tensing each area in your body and releasing it. Be aware of your head, your face, your neck, your throat, and your jaw. Breathe in deeply and allow the tension to release from these areas.

4 Move your focus down your body to your arms. Breathe in, and as you breathe out, allow the tension to release from your arms, hands, and fingers. Focus on your legs, breathe in, and as you breathe out allow the tension to release from your thighs, knees, calves, ankles, feet, and toes.

5 Focus on your back, breathing deeply into your spine, feeling the energy of your breath flowing up and down. Feel your chest expanding with each breath. Finally, focus on your baby, breathing long, slow breaths to your baby, feeling united as a family.

6 Slowly start to deepen your breath. Feel with each deep breath that you are coming closer to the surface and awakening. Keep breathing deeply until you open your eyes. Finish with a gentle stretch.

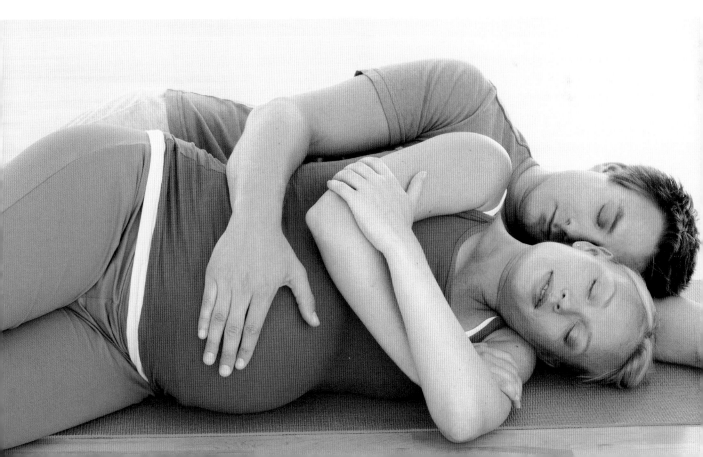

Breathing awareness

Yoga is the breath, and it is the breath that you should draw upon when giving birth to your baby. By learning to focus upon your breath, you are enabling yourself to turn inward and go to a place deep inside where you can find comfort and support.

Breathing affects the way you feel – if you breathe in a fast and furious way, your heart will beat fast, your pulse will quicken, and you will start to feel anxious and panicky. Equally, if you quieten your breath, gently working on a deep in breath and a long, slow out breath, you will begin to relax, your heart rate will slow down, and you will feel calm and more centred. This is important, because although you may not be able to change a situation, you can change your breathing pattern to alter the way you feel about it. For labour this is invaluable – a woman who can focus on her breath is able to remain calm and centred.

By breathing deeply, you are providing yourself and your baby with oxygen, and the long, slow out breath enables you to relax, producing more endorphins, which are nature's way to counter pain and stress. A long, slow out breath also makes more room for a good intake of breath. Physiologically, the breathing exercises maintain equilibrium in your body, keeping your blood pressure balanced.

Breathing exercises (or *pranayama*), are your tools. You might feel comfortable with only one or two of them, but that is fine. Practise them with awareness until they become second nature – then you will be able to use them instinctively with your chosen positions during labour and birthing. The breathing exercises fall into two groups: those that you can use during contractions in labour and birth, and those that you use to maintain peace and well-being, either between contractions or out of the birth room. You will probably have an instant liking for some of the exercises, and these will be the ones you use in labour.

Use the following pages to familiarize yourself with your breath. By being aware of your breath, you will be more observant of yourself and your body and can also recognize if you are tense or holding your breath. Once you are familiar with your breathing, you can work on lengthening your breath . Through **joined breathing** (see opposite page), your partner will also become familiar with your breath and be able to recognize any changes. He will be able to find ways to help you with your breath, so that if you feel unable to cope with a contraction, he can tell you to release your breath with a long, slow "haaa!" and help you breathe a long, slow breath until you feel you have regained control.

The exercises can be practised at any time in a quiet environment, but be aware of the following points. Unlike traditional yoga, you must breathe in through your nose and breathe out through your mouth, unless the exercise instructs you otherwise. You must sit in a comfortable position. This may be cross-legged or the **hero's pose** (see page 25). Make sure you have plenty of cushions to support you. Remember that these are sitting positions to practise breathing – you won't be using them in labour. Familiarize yourself with the exercises, and when you are confident try putting them together with the suggested labour positions – for example, walking, leaning forward on bean bags, or on all fours. Be patient, and stop if you feel breathless or unwell. Never hold your breath and don't exaggerate your in breath because this may cause you to hyperventilate, which is dangerous in pregnancy. Don't practise all the breathing exercises at once. It's too much and can make you feel unwell. Choose one or two and do them slowly and gently.

These deep breathing exercises can make you feel emotional. If this happens don't worry – take a break and try again later. If you suffer from depression, mental illness, or are taking medication, consult with your doctor before doing these exercises.

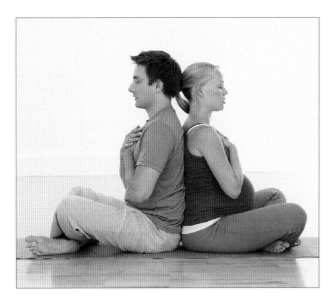

◁ Breath awareness

1 Sit comfortably and upright, either alone or back to back with your partner. Place your hands on your chest and gently take long, slow breaths, feeling the movement against your hands.

2 Place your hands on your rib cage and focus on your breath in your rib cage.

3 Place your hands on your tummy and breathe with long, slow breaths in to your tummy area. Now focus on breathing long, slow breaths only to your baby. Aim for your in breath to go as deep as it can and your out breath to last as long as possible.

Joined breathing ▷

By breathing together and touching your unborn baby, you have a chance to unite at a deep level and learn about your partner's breath.

Relax in a comfortable position with your partner so you can both place your hands over your baby, perhaps with you sitting cross-legged and your partner behind you. Breathe long, slow breaths into your hands and feel how your baby responds to the deep breathing.

TIP If you don't want to do a complete yoga sequence, try doing only breathing practices (pranayama). Start with a few minutes first thing in the morning and just before bedtime, and gradually build up the time.

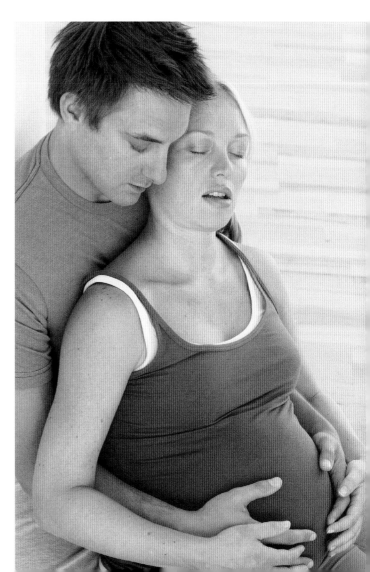

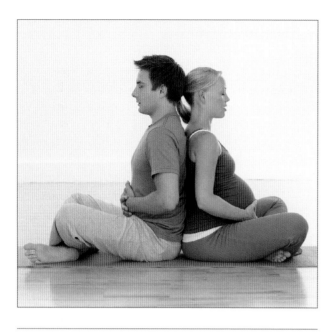

Experiment with the sound. You may be more comfortable with one sound than another.

◄ Breathing with sound

Breathing with sound will help you enter a deep level of meditation. It is useful during the first stage of labour and in giving birth.

1 Sit comfortably and upright, either alone or back to back with your partner. Begin by scrunching up your face as you breathe in and releasing tension as you breathe out with a big "ha!" breath. Gently close your eyes.

2 Breathe in deeply and on the next out breath let the sound "ahhhhh" come out. Don't rush – allow it to reach the end. Repeat three times. Breathe in again. This time let the sound "ohhhhh" come out on the out breath. Repeat three times. Breathe in and let the sound "mmmmm" escape. Repeat three times.

3 Let your breaths gently return to normal. Breathe a few long, slow breaths before opening your eyes.

Number breathing ►

Number breathing is a useful focal technique during labour, especially if you feel unable to cope.

1 Sit comfortably upright, either alone or back to back with your partner. Close your eyes, take a deep in breath and release a big out breath with a "ha!" to get rid of any tension. Focus on the flow of your in breath and your out breath. Slowly start to count your breaths, noting pauses between each breath. Breathe in for the count of 4 and out for the count of 6. If your mind wanders, bring it back to focus on your breath.

2 Repeat this five times, focusing on the numbers.

TIP If these numbers feel too much, try breathing in for 3 counts and out for 5.

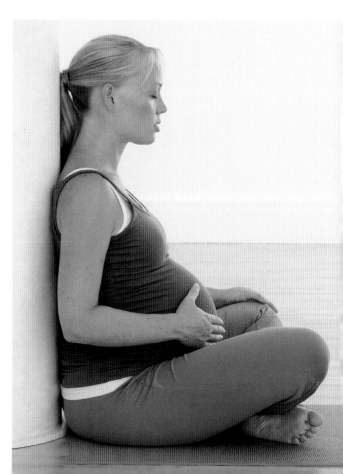

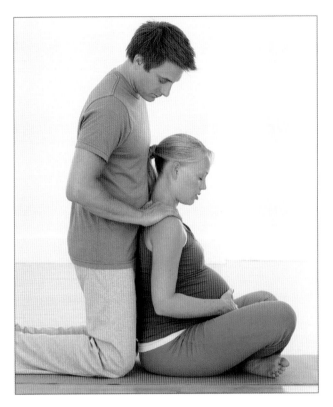

◄ **Shoulder touch**

The gentle touch and presence of your partner can be enough to help you through a difficult part of labour. This exercise can be done with your partner either kneeling or sitting on a chair behind you. Even if you are lying on your side, the gentle touch can be helpful.

1 Sit comfortably and upright, place your hands on your baby, and breathe long, slow breaths.

2 Ask your partner to place his hands lightly on your shoulders and observe your breathing. When you breathe out, he should gently press on your shoulders, being careful not to rush you or push too hard. Ask him to move his hands away from your shoulders as you breathe in. Repeat five times.

3 Now try it with sound. As you breathe out, allow a long "ahhhhh" sound to escape, which will encourage you to breathe out for longer.

Alternate nostril breathing ►

The alternate nostril breathing (*nadi shodhana*) calms the mind and promotes good sleep. Some women find it helpful in late pregnancy if they can't sleep or are worried about the birth.

1 Sit comfortably upright, either alone or back to back with your partner. Using your right hand, place your thumb over your right nostril, your first two fingers at the top of your nose. and your ring finger beside your left nostril.

2 Breathe in through your left nostril; cover your left nostril, breathe out of your right nostril. Now breathe in through your right nostril; cover your right nostril, and breathe out of your left nostril.

3 Repeat three or four times, breathing evenly.

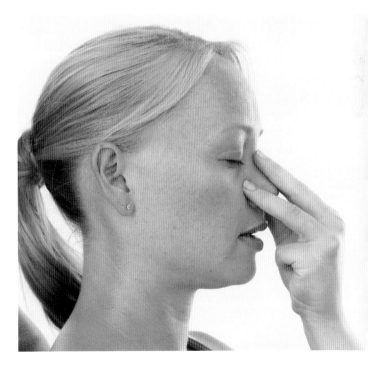

Bee breath (*Brahmari* breath) ▼

The bee breath is a "sound breath" that some women find helpful when working with contractions. It can be calming and can help insomnia and relax the body, mind, and spirit.

1 Sit comfortably upright, either alone or back to back with your partner. Close your eyes and allow your breath to gently slow down. Relax your jaw and keep your mouth soft.

2 Inhale slowly and deeply through your nostrils. As you breathe out slowly, make a humming noise like a bee for as long as the out breath lasts.

3 Repeat five or six times. Allow your breath to return to normal before slowly opening your eyes.

Hissing breath ▼

This can be used during contractions. Allow your breath to flow and follow it with your mind. The longer the out breath, the more power you'll have to help with pain.

1 Sit comfortably upright, either alone or back to back with your partner. Close your eyes and focus on your breath.

2 Hold your teeth lightly together and separate the lips, exposing the teeth. Breathe in slowly and deeply through your nose; then breathe out through your lips, producing a long, thin breath.

3 Repeat four or five times and allow your breath to return to normal.

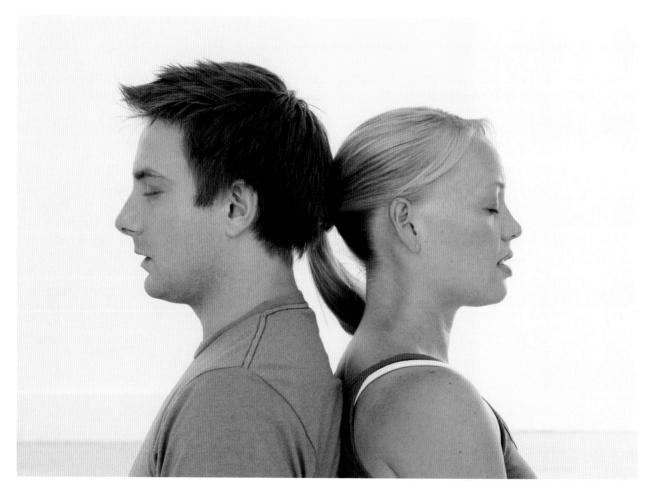

Victorious breath (*Ujjayi* breath)

Victorious breath can be used by women in labour to remain calm and centred. By focusing on the sound of the breath, you can go to a deep level of meditation. Some women are able to work with contractions by focusing entirely on this breath. Others prefer to use it between contractions to bring them back to centre.

1 Sit comfortably upright, against a wall or back to back with your partner. Close your eyes and focus on the natural rhythm of your breath.

2 Turn your awareness to the back of your throat. Breathe in, and as you breathe out contract the area at the back of your throat (glottis) by imagining that the breath is being drawn to the back of your throat. The out breath will become slower and deeper, with a soft snoring sound like a sleeping baby. The sound should be gentle and only audible to a person next to you.

3 Repeat five or six times, each time focusing on the out breath, drawing it out a little bit longer. When you finish your practice, allow your breath to return to normal and slowly open your eyes.

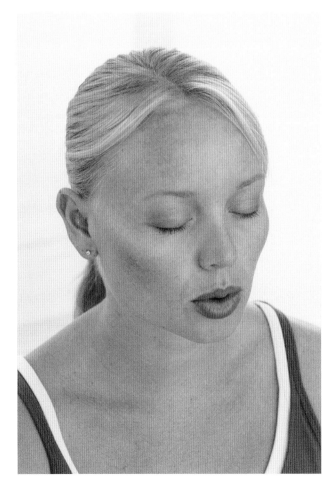

◄ Cooling breath

This breath is useful between contractions to help you replenish your energy for the next set of contractions.

1 Sit comfortably upright, either alone or back to back with your partner. Close your eyes and follow your breath's natural rhythm.

2 Roll the sides of your tongue up so that it forms a tube, or form the shape of an "O" with your mouth. Inhale and draw the breath in. At the end of the breath draw your tongue in, close your mouth, and exhale through your nose. Your breath can be long and slow or at your normal pace.

3 Repeat four to five times. When you finish allow your breath to return to normal.

TIP Sometimes the cooling breath exercise can make you thirsty. If you plan to use this breath in labour, have water to hand and sip it as needed.

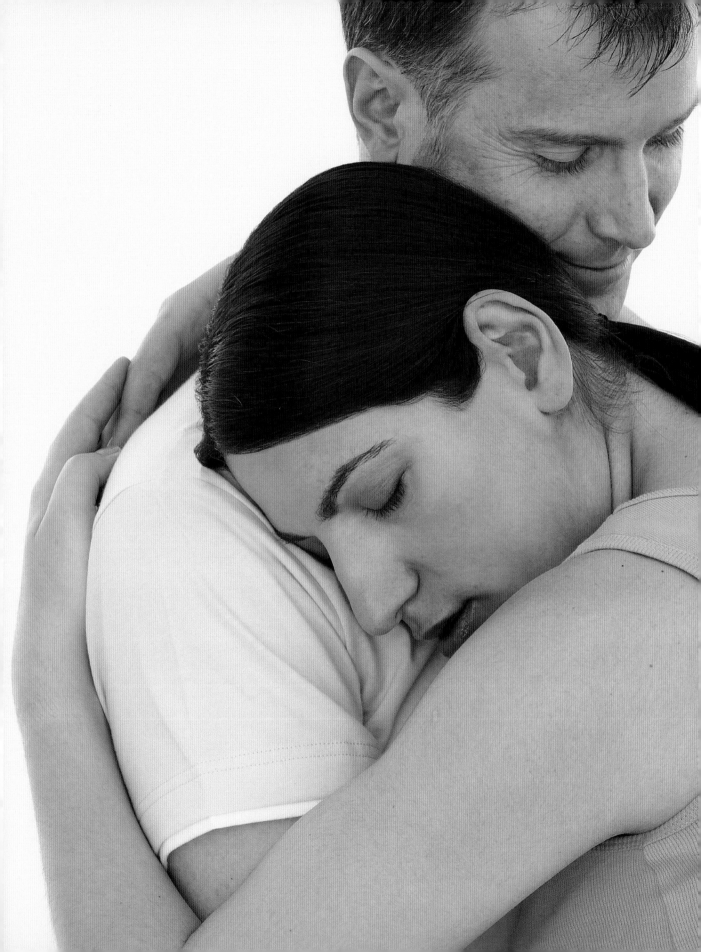

The first stage

Just as you breathe in and breathe out
Sometimes you're ahead and other times behind.
Sometimes you're strong and other times weak.
Tao Te Ching, Chapter 29

The first stage of labour

This section looks at how you can recognize the first signs of labour, and how you can use yoga movements and breathing to focus on your contractions. It also explores the roles of hormones, and it explains the different positions helpful for you during labour and how to use breathing and massage to support you in hospital and at home.

Every woman experiences labour in a different way, but there are definite signs that indicate that labour is imminent or has already begun. If you are unsure, always seek medical advice.

- You will experience labour contractions that have a rhythmic quality, with each contraction gradually building and peaking, then fading. They will increase in intensity over time.
- The contractions will require all your concentration, and you will need to rest between them.
- Labour contractions are sometimes felt as a minor backache, with regular bouts of stronger back pain.
- Occasionally the membrane leaks or breaks, which is often referred to as your "waters breaking".
- Contractions can start immediately but often take hours to become established.

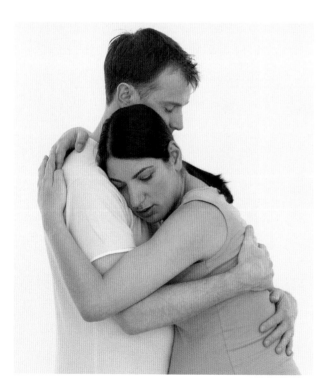

The classic labour starts when you have regular contractions, 2–3 minutes apart and 20–30 seconds long. The contractions will become steadily more frequent and of longer duration, until at the end of the first stage of labour, when the cervix is almost fully open, and they are only 30 seconds apart and 60–90 seconds long. However, few women have such a textbook labour and there is great variety in the pattern of rhythms. The length of the first stage of labour varies, but it is between 8 and 16 hours on average for a first birth.

The onset of labour can be exciting and frightening. Your safety and the safety of your baby is the priority – you will need to place trust in your medical carers and in your own abilities to give birth instinctively.

THE MECHANICS OF LABOUR

By understanding the physiology of labour, you can make your environment more conducive to birth so that you are able to turn to your yoga, breathing, and partner for support.

You were born equipped with the innate instinctive behaviours that are designed to help you reproduce. The controlling centres for these behaviours are in the primitive part of the brain that controls urges such as hunger, thirst, stress, anger, and sexual behaviour. Most of the time, the circumstances that trigger the "fight and flight" mechanisms of survival are separate from those that encourage us to reproduce. However, during labour the two drives become interconnected; you as the mother, while following your reproductive instincts, will feel vulnerable, and a successful birth will depend on you being protected. It is the interplay of the mechanisms of survival and reproduction that shape much of the physiology of labour and birth.

The mechanisms are governed by several hormones such as oxytocin, adrenaline, and endorphins. You cannot control their release because they are secreted automatically. The flow of labour is controlled by oxytocin, the "love hormone". Oxytocin is needed to stimulate contractions. The more loved, looked-after, and safe you feel, the higher your oxytocin levels and the more effective your contractions will be. The action of oxytocin is affected by adrenaline. When adrenaline is produced – because you are scared, or due to a change in your environment such as lack of privacy, feeling cold, or bright lights – your contractions may stop, be less effective, or feel more painful.

It is important to remember that all women are different, and what might be a comfort to some might be an annoyance to others. For example, classical music might be an oxytocin enhancer for you, but it might produce adrenaline in someone else. This is important for your birth partner to understand, because he or she can provide the right environment that will help to increase your levels of oxytocin and endorphins. Endorphins will help to protect you from excessive pain during labour, and produce an altered state that allows you to turn inward and focus.

MOVEMENTS AND POSITIONS FOR THE FIRST STAGE

If you are already in active labour, the movements on the following pages will encourage you to move around by walking and moving your hips, which can help speed things up. There are also positions to help you when you need to relax between contractions, as you will need the stamina to continue throughout. As the labour progresses, you may find leaning forward onto a chair helpful, using your partner to support you. The stronger your contractions are, the more you may wish to be close to the ground, perhaps on all fours and resting forward on a bean bag between contractions. The key is to combine these positions and movements with your breath – your out breath is the real tool for controlling pain.

WHAT'S GOING ON?

During the first stage of labour the cervix dilates from closed to open (0–10cm/0–4in). Your baby moves down deeper into the pelvis, rotating slowly into the widest part of the pelvis as he or she descends. As your baby's head descends it exerts pressure on the cervix, assisting dilation.

The dilating uterus pulls up around the head like a glove as it passes down the pelvic canal. By the time you are fully dilated, it will have drawn up around your baby's head as far as the ears and opened wide enough for your baby's body to pass through. During early dilation (0–4cm/0–1½in), the cervix softens, shortens (effaces), and begins to dilate. As dilation reaches 4–5cm (1½–2in), labour enters the accelerated phase. The contractions will be stronger, closer together, and will need concentration. You will feel the need to rest more between contractions, and you will want to turn in and focus on the activity in your body.

BREATHING FOR THE FIRST STAGE OF LABOUR

Centre yourself by focusing on your breath. When you need to deepen your breath, focus on expanding your in breath and lengthening your out breath. Try any of the breathing exercises such as breathing with sound, number breathing, hissing breath, shoulder touch with sound, or victorious breath (see pages 32–37). Remember to keep your shoulders relaxed, jaw loose, and relax your body between contractions.

Helpful hints for the first stage

WHAT MUM MIGHT FEEL AND CAN DO

Some women describe the first signs of labour as not at all painful, only uncomfortable, while others find the pain difficult to cope with.

- If the pains are only uncomfortable and lack intensity you can continue with your normal activity, perhaps taking a walk or getting some sleep.

- When you feel your contractions are demanding all your focus, if you have chosen to have your baby in hospital, it may be time to go.

- Try to keep refuelled with regular snacks such as cereal bars or sip a sweet drink.

- Use the positions and breathing suggested in this section. Evidence suggests that staying active at the early stage encourages your cervix to dilate more quickly – but don't exhaust yourself.

- It's normal to feel anxious in a hospital environment. Try to stay focused on your prepared breathing, using sound breathing (see page 34) or the number breath (see page 34).

- Try to take each contraction at a time – fearful anticipation of increasing pain may slow down labour.

- Immersion in warm water once in active labour (when dilated 4cm/1½in plus) can speed things up and might help you to relax. Make use of a birth pool if available or use the bath or shower.

- Above all, stay positive – labour may seem long but you will soon be welcoming your baby. (This applies to your partner too.)

WHAT DAD MIGHT FEEL AND CAN DO

Your support as a birth partner is vital. During early labour, ensure your partner is well fuelled and encourage her to move around, but don't get her tired.

- Make sure she's warm and that she has sweet drinks and some refuelling snacks.

- When you get to hospital (if you have chosen to have your baby in hospital) your partner may feel anxious. Keep her stress levels down.

- Encourage her to empty her bladder. A full bladder slows down labour.

- Respect her privacy – she may feel more comfortable with her underwear on, until the birth. Keep the room dark if she finds this reassuring.

- Keep the room familiar and homely, perhaps with her favourite music, scents, or pillow.

- Once a comfortable position is found, use it until she signals that it is no longer helping her relax. Breathe with her if she can't cope with the contractions.

- If labour is slow you may find it helpful to change the mood and scene. Take her for a walk or move her to another room. Be encouraging and don't hurry her.

- Make sure she feels compatible with her midwife. You can ask for another midwife if needed.

- Think of yourself too – you will be no use to her if you are drained. Have a drink and a stretch and make sure you eat enough to keep up your energy.

Movements and positions for the first stage

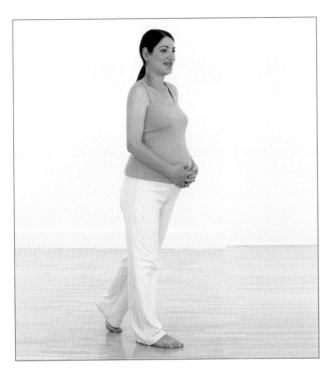

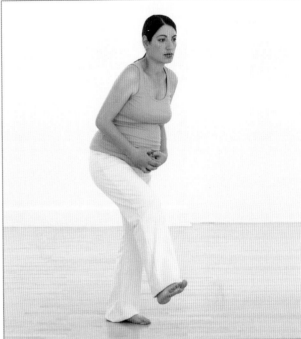

Walking ▲

Try walking in the first stage of labour. Walking can shorten labour and increase the efficiency of the contractions.

1 Begin walking gently, making sure your shoulders and jaw are relaxed. As the contraction comes, breathe out with a long, slow "ahhhh" sound. Avoid holding your breath and don't exhaust yourself. Rest between contractions, either by **leaning into a wall** (see page 44) or **sitting astride a chair** (see page 45).

TIP Rest between contractions and don't exhaust yourself. You can alternate between camel walking, leaning into the wall, and sitting astride a chair.

Camel walking ▲

This sequence may be effective for trying to speed up a labour, especially if the baby is in the *occipito-posterior* position (see glossary).

1 Begin by walking normally. Check that your jaw is relaxed and your teeth are not clenched. Then gently lean forward and peel your feet off the ground, picking one foot up at a time. You don't have to exaggerate the movement.

2 Synchronize your breath with the movement. Breathe out long, slow breaths and try **breathing with sound** (see page 34) as the contractions come. Make the sounds "ahhh–ohhh–mmmm".

Leaning into a wall ▶

The support of a wall is helpful, either at home or in hospital. Leaning into the wall can be used as a means to rest between contractions.

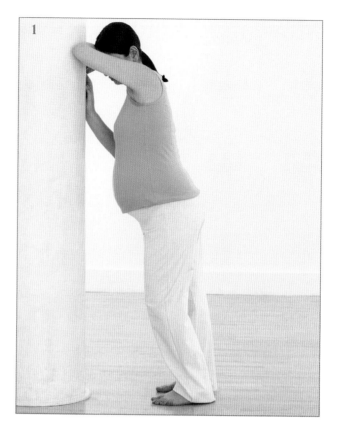

1 To help cope with your contractions you can try hiding your face with your hands, moving your hips in small circles, and using the **breathing with sound** (see page 34).

2 Your partner can support you with massage by using long, slow strokes from the top of your spine all the way down to your ankles.

3 If you have a backache in labour, your partner can gently place the balls of his hands on your lower back as you breathe out. You may just like the warmth or may prefer some pressure.

4 If you are shaky, ask your partner to gently massage your legs with long, downward strokes. Make sure your partner bends his knees when giving you a massage to protect his back.

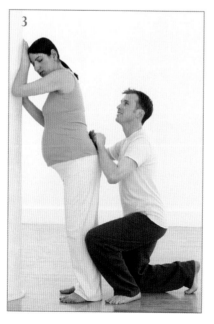

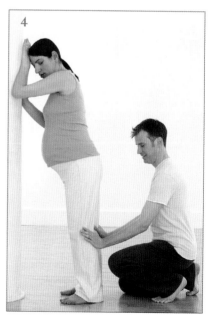

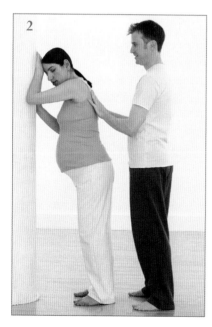

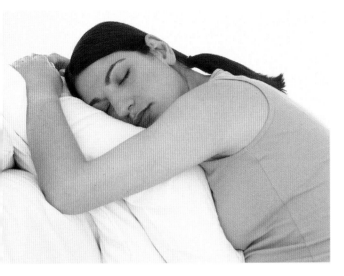

◄ Using a chair and a bed for support

As you have contractions, the uterus tilts forward, so any forward leaning position helps your contractions to work more efficiently and less painfully. You can sit on the edge of a chair, or perhaps you may prefer the support of the bed as you lean forward.

Sit forward on a chair and rest your head onto the bed. The bed should be at the same level. If it helps, place cushions under your feet and cushions under your head. You may want a blanket over your head to maintain privacy and security and enhance oxytocin production (see glossary).

Sitting astride a chair ▼

As labour progresses, some women prefer to sit.

1 Sit astride a chair, facing its back. Make sure there are plenty of cushions to rest your head against.

2 Your partner can gently massage your back if this helps, from the shoulders to the lower back. Try to synchronize the strokes with your breathing sounds of "ahhh–ohhh–mmmm".

3 If the contractions are difficult, ask your partner to try the **shoulder touch** technique (see page 35). If you are tense or panicked, let out a big sigh or "aaah" breathe. Your partner should observe your breath, and breath with you if it helps.

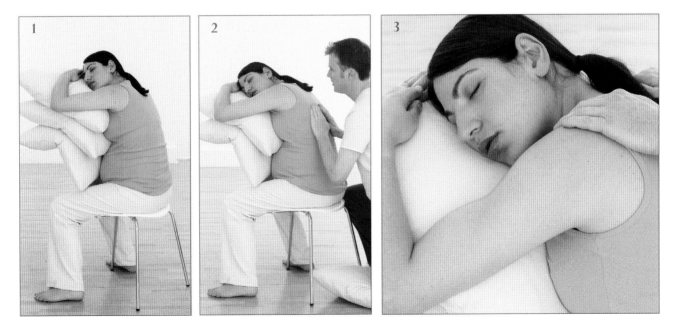

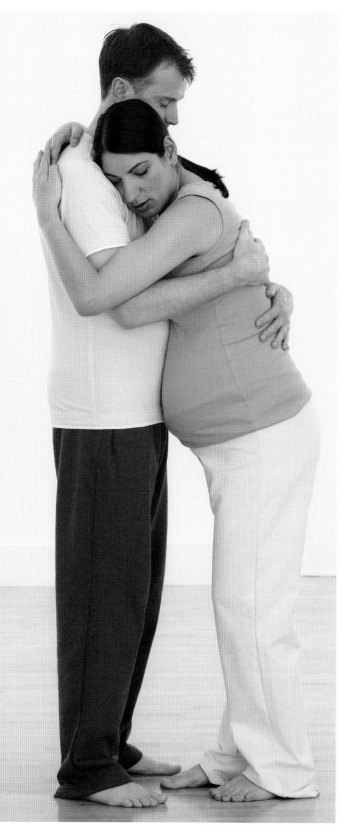

◄ Couple's embrace

Sometimes you will be too tired to move around but will want to remain upright. This embrace allows you to be supported physically and emotionally by your partner. This intimacy can keep your oxytocin levels high, encouraging effective contractions.

1 Stand in the arms of your partner as if you are doing a slow dance, leaning into and embracing him. You can turn your head into his shoulders.

2 When you feel comfortable, gently move your hips in a rhythmic way. You can use **breathing with sound** (see page 34) to help.

TIP You may be panicked or not coping too well, but you may prefer not to be touched. If this is the case, your birth partner can look you in the eyes and breathe with you, using **breathing with sound** (see page 34).

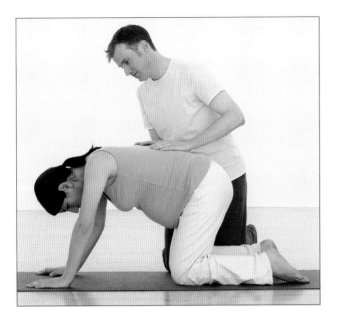

◄ On all fours

As labour progresses, many women prefer to be closer to the ground to turn inward and concentrate on the demands of the contractions.

Gently move your hips in a circle, focusing on the "ahhh–ohhh–mmmm" breaths. Moving your pelvis rhythmically during contractions – either rocking to and fro from side to side or in a slow circle – will aid the dilation of your cervix, the descent of your baby, and help dissipate the pain. You can put cushions under your knees if you need to.

Resting forward on a bean bag ▼

You can rest between contractions on a bean bag, cushion, or against a bed.

1 Make sure you are leaning forwards – any forward leaning position assists contractions, making them quicker and less painful.

2 Your partner can massage you in all positions by placing his hands on your lower back or using long, slow strokes down your body, synchronized with your breath.

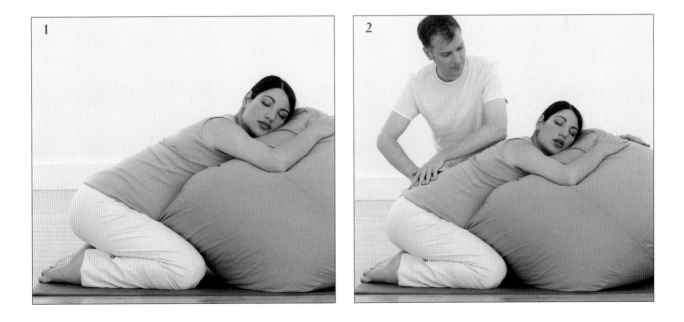

What if I'm in hospital?

You will be able to walk in hospital. Try strolling up and down the ward or around the room. This is a good way to speed up labour. Between contractions if you want to rest try **couple's embrace** (see page 46).

If you feel tired, try **using a chair and a bed for support** (see page 45). Focus on your breath.

If labour is slow and you need some privacy, you can continue your labour in the toilet. You can take your partner with you. Remember he can massage your back or breathe with you. Bring your cushions.

If you have to be on the bed for whatever reason, try going **on all fours** (see page 47) and circling your hips, use your "ahhh–ohhh–mmmm" breath. Rest forward against the bed head.

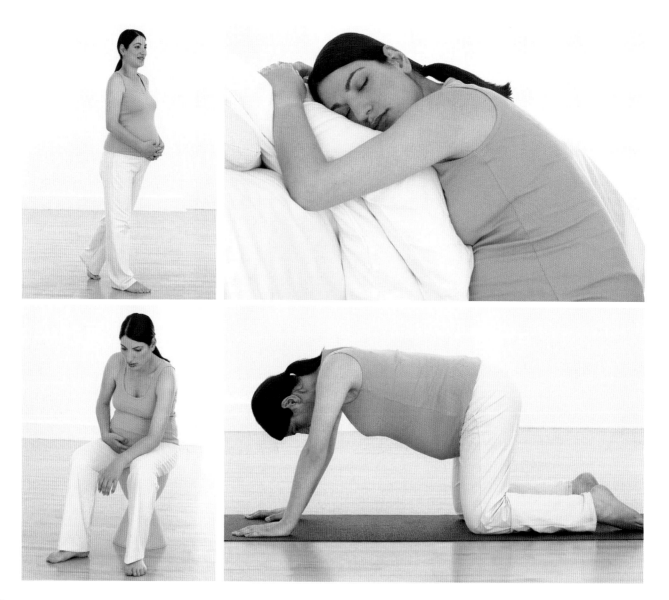

What if I'm at home?

You can use the space of your home to walk around. If you want to speed up labour you can walk up and down stairs, or into the garden if you have one. Remember your long, slow breaths.

You may want to try **leaning into a wall** (see page 44). Remember your partner can massage you if you want, synchronizing the massage with your breath.

At home you can make the most of your comforts. Why not light a candle in the room, play your favourite music, sit on your stool under the shower, or maybe have a bath? These can all help relieve pain.

You may feel comfortable to be on the floor **on all fours** (see page 47), moving your hips with the support of your partner massaging your back.

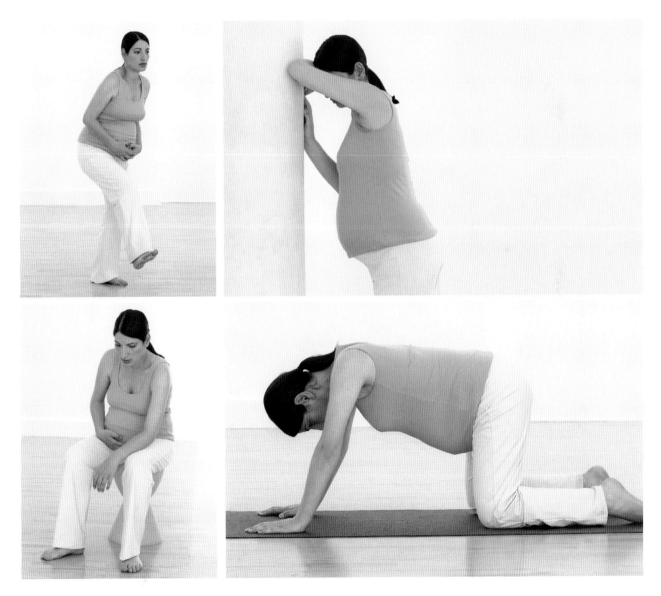

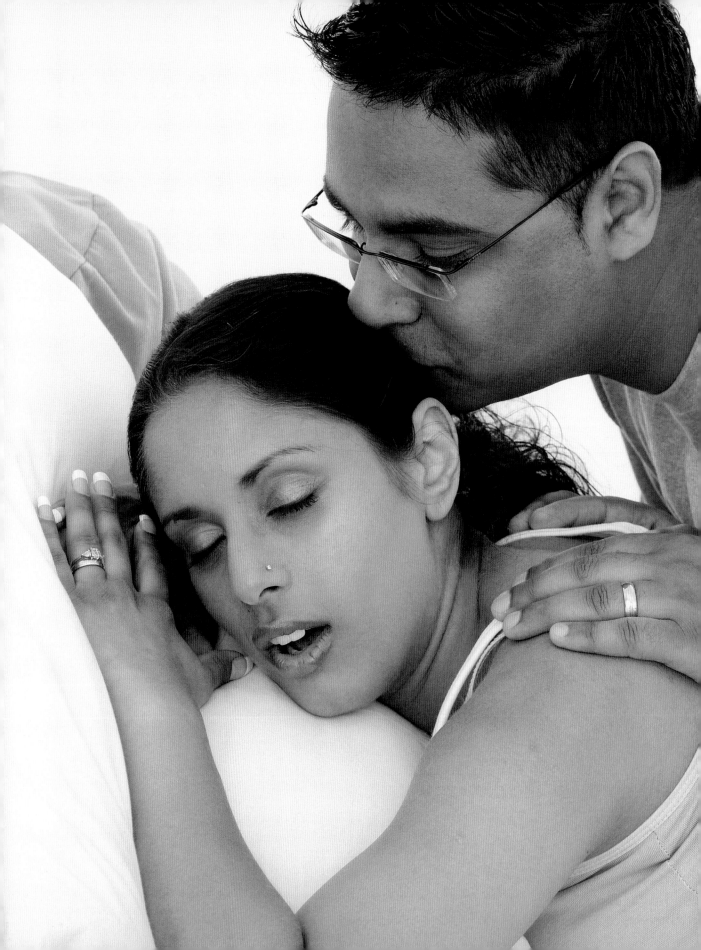

The transition

The individual soul is
unbreakable and insoluble.

Bhagavad Gita, Chapter 2, Verse 24

The transition stage of labour

The term "transition" is used to describe the last and most intense part of the first stage of labour – when the baby begins the descent into the vagina, with perhaps the onset of the urge to bear down. It can last only a few minutes or go on for half an hour or so. This section explains how to recognize when you are in transition and how you can use yoga, breathing, and your partner's support.

Transition contractions need to be long and strong to get the cervix to open those last few centimetres. There is little or no respite between the contractions and many women say this is the hardest part of labour.

Some women become distressed and weepy during this time, and they may feel despair, nauseous, shaky, and out of control. They may also make lots of noise, cry out for help, or panic-stricken. Others become uncommunicative and silent. Sometimes women become irritable or aggressive during transition, so birth partners should be prepared for verbal or even physical abuse! Women who wanted physical contact from their partners may suddenly demand "don't touch me". Another sign of transition is talk about dying: "I'm dying!" or "Let me die!". This is another symptom of the sudden rush of adrenaline that sets the "fetus ejection reflex" in motion, which is needed to bring your baby into the world (see glossary).

TRANSITION AND PAIN RELIEF

When contractions really hurt it becomes harder to sustain your resolve to avoid drugs for pain relief. This is a phase of labour in which even the women who have birth plans committed to avoiding pain relief may demand an epidural. However, if you have come this far without pain relief it might be a pity to give up when you are so nearly there, particularly as using drugs at this stage might result in difficulties during the second stage of labour. It is well worth "hanging in there" and relying on help from your birth partner.

Your birth partner may guess that you are in transition but it may not have occurred to you that you are close to giving birth to your baby. It can help if your partner tells you that this is a passing phase and

BELOW You will need the support of your birth partner more than ever during this stage.

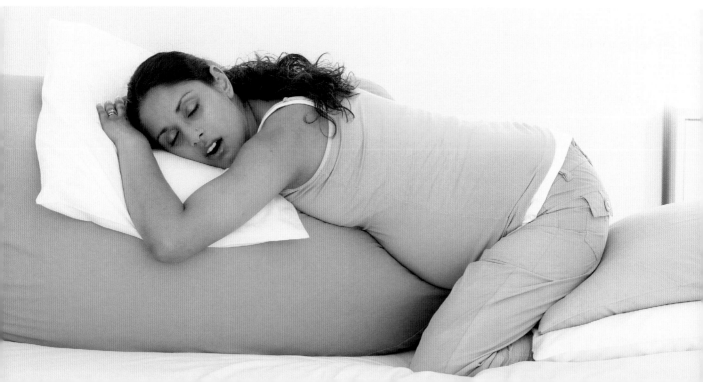

is probably as bad as it is going to get. It won't be long before you will be able to push and the contractions are likely to become shorter and less painful, with much longer pain-free rests between them. It can be distressing for your partner to see you in so much pain and sometimes a woman will accept pain-relieving drugs because her partner can't bear it. No matter how distressed your partner may be feeling at your pain, if he or she knows you want to do your best to avoid using drugs, they won't mention them.

Pain does not need to be modified with the use of drugs. Simple non-pharmaceutical methods such as yoga practices and breathing can be effective in helping you cope with transition. If the people around you remain positive and encouraging, you are more likely to have the courage to continue. Once the cervix is fully dilated (10cm/4in) the labour will change. You should feel relief and excitement as you shift from the passive surrender experienced during the dilation contractions to the more active participation in giving birth to your baby. This is a turning point in labour and is often accompanied by a sudden burst of energy, optimism, and enthusiasm.

POSITIONS FOR THE TRANSITION STAGE
The kneeling positions in this section are often the most popular to use in transition, when women tend to like being close to the ground. Remember to use cushions, bean bags, and blankets for comfort. Allow yourself to sink into a deep inner relaxation. It can be helpful to take sips of water or suck on chips of ice. Women often experience a primitive sucking reflex during labour. If you have a long transition, try changing positions occasionally. You may want to walk (see page 43) or to remain upright, leaning into the wall (see page 44). You may want to try sitting at the edge of a chair (see page 45) or toilet, or if this gets tough, try lying on your side, well propped-up with cushions.

WHAT'S GOING ON?

Your contractions are coming fast and furious with short intervals between them. They can arrive every two minutes and last one-and-a-half to one-and-three-quarter minutes, leaving only fifteen seconds or so to rest between, making them feel continuous. Your cervix is probably 8–9cm (3–3½ in) dilated, but the last centimetre (½ in) may be slow to dilate. You are on the bridge between the last dilating contractions and the beginning of the bearing down and second stage of labour. As your baby descends a little farther in the pelvic canal, the uterus draws up around the baby's head. He or she is beginning to move out of the uterus, ready to be born.

BREATHING TIPS FOR TRANSITION

You can use your breathing to help you relax (see pages 32–7). Try the sound breath, focusing on extending the out breath with your sound. Or you can combine the victorious breath and the hissing breath to counter the pain. Because of the intensity of transition, now is the time when your partner's support is needed most. He can try the shoulder touch with the sound breath. Or he can breathe with you, using the number breath.

Helpful hints for the transition stage

WHAT MUM MIGHT FEEL AND CAN DO

- You may feel distressed, weepy, nauseous, shaky, out of control, or silent. Stay positive – you are at the hardest point and it will only get better.

- Don't worry about what people will think – do what you need to do. You may want to be alone or just with your partner – it's your birth.

- Turn to your breath. Sound breath will help. Extend your out breath as you focus on it.

- Try to rest between contractions, even if just for a few moments. Let go completely. You may want to try victorious breath or cooling breath (see page 37) between your contractions.

- Wear whatever you feel most at home in. Any familiar clothes will help you in labour. You may even want to take your clothes off.

- Some women can feel sick or get mild diarrhoea. Don't worry as this is normal and your midwife will support you.

- You may have some backache as your baby descends, ready to be born. Try moving your hips in a circle, using your "ahhh–ohhh–mmmm" breath. Warm water and massage may help.

- If you are on the bed and feel tired, try to avoid lying on your back. Try to lie on your side, or even better, rest forward on a bean bag or bed head.

- Most hospital beds are adjustable. They can be lowered and the back can be raised. Why not go to the hospital beforehand and check it out?

- Above all, remain positive. You are soon going to meet your baby.

WHAT DAD MIGHT FEEL AND CAN DO

- Accept and understand her tears and moods, yet stay calm yourself.

- Anchor her as much as possible with your hands, your eyes, your voice, and your reassuring presence.

- Create more privacy if possible and keep disturbances to a minimum.

- Help her to change position if progress in transition is slow. She may find being on her hands and knees the most comfortable position, but being upright might help with dilation.

- Breathe with her and help her back to deep rhythmic breathing whenever possible. Try the sound breath "ahhh–ohhh–mmmm" or breathing with numbers.

- Make sure her shoulders and neck are loose and relaxed and that she is not gritting her teeth.

- Try every comfort measure you can think of, maybe massage, breathing, a story, or reminding her of something lovely you did together.

- Immersion in warm water, a shower, a bath or birth pool, could help alleviate some of the pain.

- Remind her to try the knee to chest position (see page 30) during a few contractions if she has the urge to push before her midwife says she is ready.

- Make sure she has a drink to sip, or ice to suck.

- If your partner has backache, try back massage or put warm, wet towels on her lower back.

- Stay calm and positive and tell her she can do it.

Positions for the transition stage

On all fours ▼

For your transition stage, you can go on your hands and knees on the floor, on the bed, or wherever it feels comfortable. Your partner can make sounds with you, focusing on a long, slow out breath. Remember to relax your jaw and avoid gritting your teeth. You may want to rest forward and relax on a bean bag between contractions (see page 47).

TIP Keep energized by sipping sweet drinks, herb tea with honey, or fruit juice. You may prefer to suck cool water from a sponge. Your partner can wipe your forehead with a cool, wet cloth.

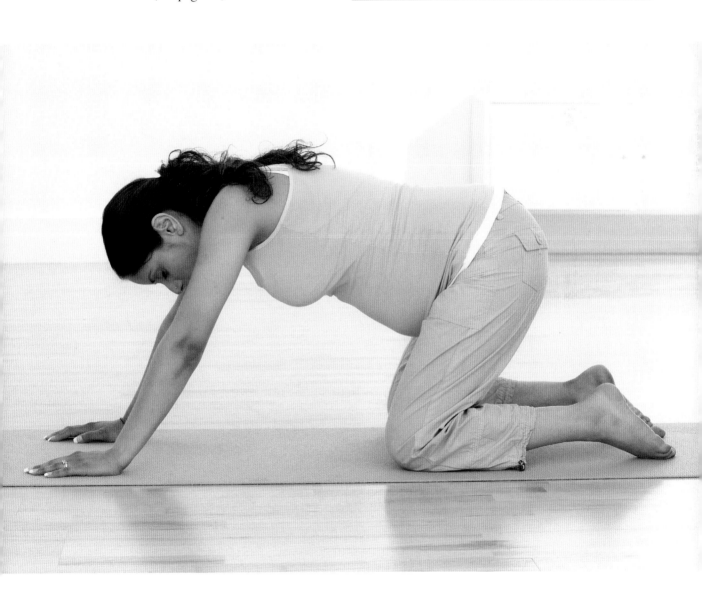

Upright kneeling position ▼

1 Try resting forward on bean bags or cushions against the bed head. This will allow you to be supported and comfortable. Make sure that your body is upright to allow gravity to assist you, and to help you use the powerful energy of the contractions within your body.

2 Rest forward between contractions. You could use a more horizontal kneeling position if you want to slow things down a little. The more horizontal your body, the slower the contractions become because the downward force of gravity weakens. Remember to use your sound or number breath.

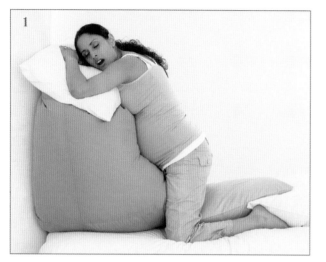

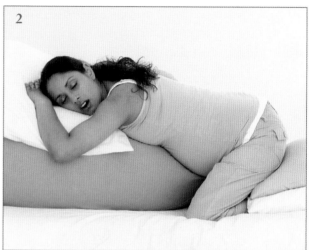

Upright kneeling position ▶ on a sofa

The sofa is a comfortable place to kneel. Make sure you have plenty of support, and that your body is upright. Your partner could place a warm, wet towel on your back to help with backache during labour.

TIP Making sure that the upper part of your body is higher than the lower part of your body will contribute to more effective and efficient contractions.

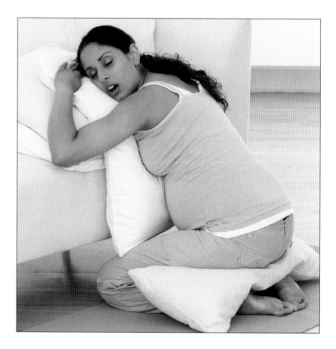

Kneeling forward with head in ▶ partner's lap

If you want to be near the floor, try resting forward into your partner's lap while he sits on a chair.

Place a cushion on his lap so you are supported. Keep your knees slightly apart and lean forward, with your back upright (not rounded). Try putting pillows under your feet and between your buttocks and your legs. If you are finding labour difficult, allow your partner to bring you back to centre with a big "haa!" breath, and then breathe long, slow breaths together.

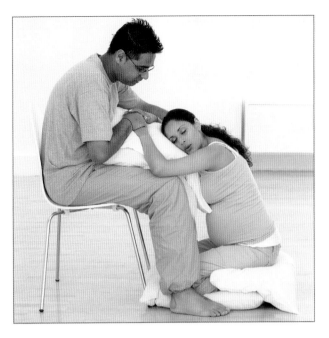

Lying on your side ▼

If you are tired and feel unable to carry on, try lying on your left side. This is preferable to a semi-reclining position or lying down. Make sure your body is well propped up by cushions and perhaps with a pillow under one knee. You can rest here between contractions and go **on all fours** (see page 55) when you have your contractions.

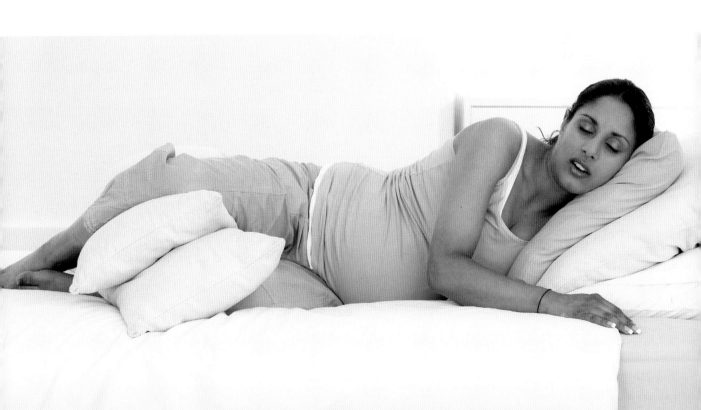

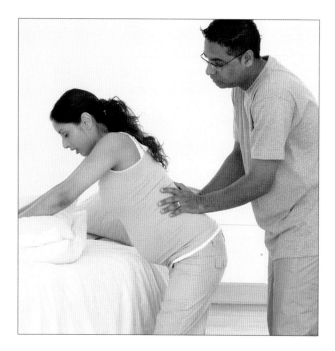

◄ Leaning onto the bed

If you preferred walking during the first stage of labour you may like to remain upright throughout. You can lean forward onto the bed, especially if it's a hospital room. Your partner can massage you, doing long strokes all the way down your body, or you may prefer the pressure of the ball of his hands on your lower back as in **leaning into a wall** (see page 44). Remember to breathe out a long breath as he massages you.

TIP Walking and stopping to lean forward during contractions can help speed up labour but avoid exhausting yourself.

Knee to chest position ► ("braking position")

The knee to chest position brings your baby's head down away from the cervix. This will help reduce the intensity of contractions in a fast labour, or if there is a premature urge to push in transition. This is also called the "braking position" because it can be used to slow down labour.

Gently place your bottom up in the air and your head down. Have a rest from the deep breathing and blow through your mouth as if you are trying to blow out a candle. This keeps the breathing superficial and avoids the need to push if it's too early. Your midwife will guide you.

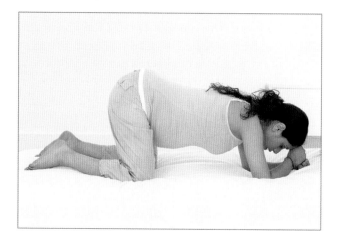

What if I'm in hospital?

In hospital you may be able to adjust the bed – most can be lowered and the bed head can be raised. Use the **upright kneeling position** (see page 56) on the bed. You can move your hips in a circle and focus on your sound breath, using long, slow breaths. Use **lying on your side** (see page 57) if you are tired and need rest. You can always get onto your hands and knees on the bed and move your hips in a circular motion. Try breathing with sound (see page 34) or number breath (see page 34).

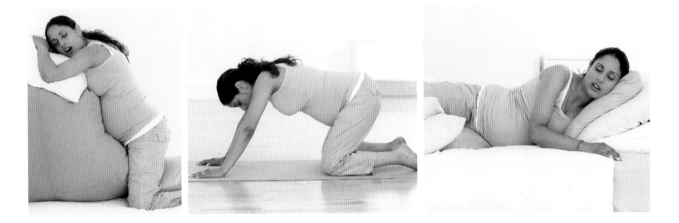

What if I'm at home?

Try the **upright kneeling position on a sofa** (see page 56), which can be helpful because you can move your hips rhythmically with support. It is also useful if you have other children sleeping in the bedrooms. Your partner can massage your back or use warm, wet towels.

You can use the **kneeling forward with head in partner's lap** posture (see page 57) to stay close to the ground. You can remain in this position for the birth, just going up onto your knees for more help from gravity. Your partner can encourage and breathe with you.

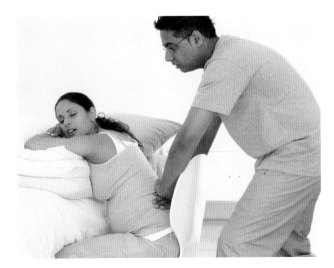
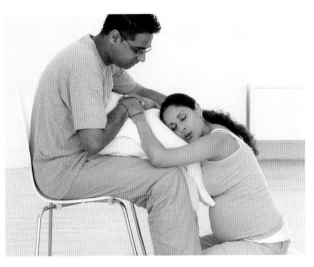

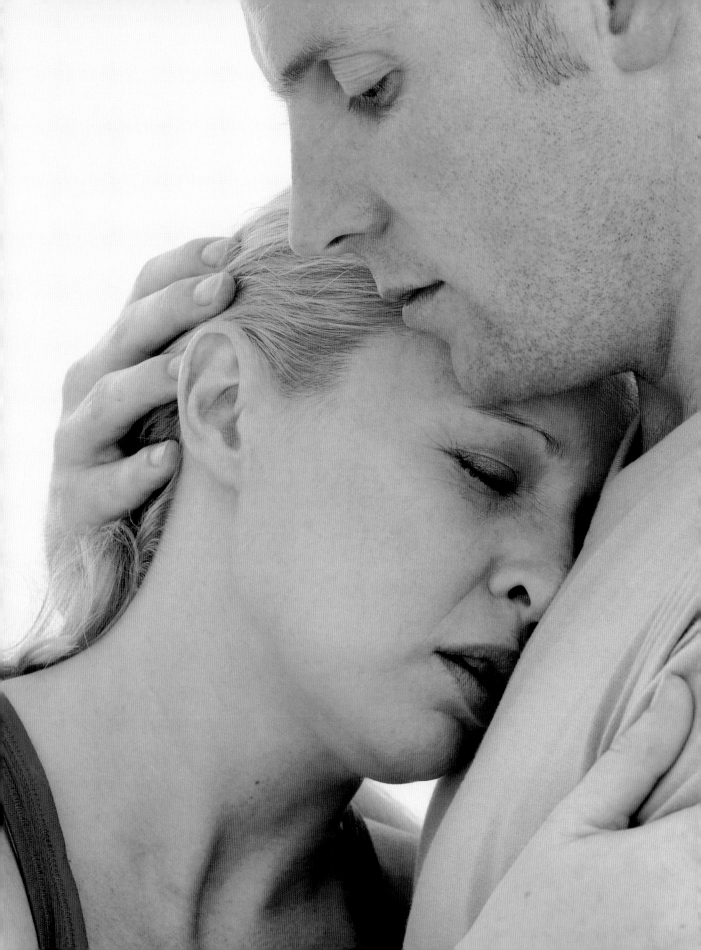

The birth

Let your body, carrying a body, bring
blessing to us and safety to you.

Rig Veda, Chapter 10, Hymn 56

Preparing for the birth

Giving birth can be described as the best part of labour. Your baby is about to arrive and anticipation is building. The rewards for all the effort will soon be realized. You may also feel a mixture of excitement and exhaustion, amazement and anxiety. This is the brief bridge between pregnancy and motherhood, the "rite of passage" into parenting.

Once the cervix is fully dilated there is often a lull when the contractions become much milder or stop altogether for a while. Midwives will recognize this as the latent, or hidden, phase of the second part of labour. This interval gives you the opportunity to relax and gather your strength prior to giving birth. This does not mean that there is a need to intervene with syntocin (see glossary) to stimulate contractions artificially. Try to make the most of the break and be patient – the active phase of the birth will get underway once the uterus and your baby are ready.

When the contractions pick up again, muscles of the uterus will be contracting to bring about a strong expulsive force that will push the baby out through the dilated cervix and down the birth canal. The force of the contractions may be powerful enough to give birth to your baby without any additional effort from

you, but usually women have an overwhelming urge to bear down and push with the contractions.

Feel confident that you will do the right thing during the birth of your baby. Any of the positions that you have used and felt comfortable with in the first stage of labour may continue to help you. Alternatively, you may find new upright positions more effective. From whatever position you are in, your partner should help you into the upright position with minimal disturbance so that gravity can assist you in giving birth. If the first stage of labour has gone on a long time, you may feel anxious that you will be too worn out to handle the birth itself. However, this is unlikely provided you are well nourished and hydrated. Even after a long first stage you will usually have new excitement and optimism with the onset of birth. Together with your partner's support, accompanied by your yoga and breathing, you will find the strength to breathe your way through birth.

HOSPITAL BIRTHS
Don't be forced by hospital staff to get up onto the bed at this point. This is an outmoded practice, except when a ventouse or forceps are needed to assist the birth. Your midwife will monitor how well your baby is doing by listening to its heart after each contraction. There should be no need to hurry, provided you are both well. Left to herself, a woman will often naturally take several breaths during each second stage contraction and give a number of little pushes with each exhalation. If you are comfortable to continue your breathing exercises you can do so during the birth. Sometimes if your midwife detects

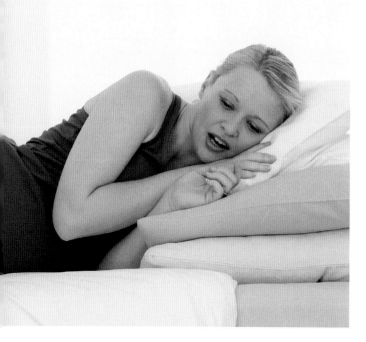

LEFT Contractions during birth may feel different in character from earlier contractions and you may make different sounds.

that your baby is in distress, she may ask you to drop your chin onto your chest, hold your breath, and push. Follow this advice if it becomes necessary to do so.

In 1996 the World Health Organization (WHO) – which has a primary responsibility for international health matters and public health – issued a report that made recommendations about birth practices. It highlighted practices that are "clearly harmful or ineffective and should be eliminated" such as the routine use of lithotomy positions, with or without stirrups, and the use of the supine position during labour. It also commended practices that are "demonstrably useful and should be encouraged" such as freedom in position and movement throughout labour and encouragement of non-supine positions.

BIRTHING CONTRACTIONS AND PUSHING

There can be a variable amount of push between the birthing contractions. One may be long and powerful, while the next is short and mild. Listen to the messages coming from your body and match the amount of effort you put into bearing down to the force of each contraction.

Your baby's head will likely descend little by little with each contraction but then slide back up the birth canal in the interval between. This may make you feel that your baby has changed its mind and wants to go back into the womb! This is normal and once your baby's head has crowned it won't slip back any more. The intense stretching and burning sensation as the head crowns is a signal to stop pushing. You may be told to stop pushing but pant to birth the head slowly and prevent tearing. When contractions are powerful and painful it is natural to hold back a little. Fear of being stretched can have the effect of creating more muscular tension. If you let go and relax the pain can be less. Your partner can encourage you to relax your face, jaw, throat, and pelvic floor. Breathe out through a relaxed open mouth and breathe your baby out.

WHAT'S GOING ON?

The second stage of labour begins when the cervix is completely dilated at 10cm (4in) and your baby's head has moved into the birth canal. He or she will gradually stretch the vaginal opening until the head crowns, and your baby's head will appear through your vagina just prior to the birth. During the birth your baby's head will emerge first, followed by the shoulders, one at a time, then the rest of his or her body.

The contractions are often shorter than transition stage contractions and there are longer rests between them. The expulsive reflex is completely involuntary – it may come quickly or it make take a while to start. There is usually a tremendous urge to bear down. However, this reflex might be absent if your baby is lying posterior, or if his or her head is slightly at a slant. Your midwife will be able to advise you what is happening, and don't be afraid to ask.

BREATHING TIPS FOR GIVING BIRTH

You will instinctively find your own way to breathe during birthing. Sound works well, so focus on your deep breath as you feel a contraction coming on and release an "ahhh" sound as you exhale. This will help you let go and relax, as well as help with pain. You will probably feel powerful needs to bear down and an uncontrollable urge to push down at the peak of each contraction. Follow your body's natural instincts, but don't hold your breath because this reduces the oxygen supply to you and your baby. As your baby's head crowns try not to push too hard. You can pant or try shallow out breaths that are less tiring.

Helpful hints for the birth

WHAT MUM MIGHT FEEL AND CAN DO

- You will find that your contractions change their nature. When you have an urge to bear down, try pushing on the ground or onto a chair.

- You don't need to go into your birthing position until your baby's head has crowned. You don't even need to take your underwear off until then.

- Try releasing your breath and making loud sounds – this will help you to relax.

- If it takes a long time for your baby to descend into the pelvis, a supported squat may speed things up.

- Try upright positions for the birth. With gravity's help your baby will be born quicker.

- Avoid lying on your back as this will be like giving birth uphill. As an alternative, go onto your side.

- Perineal massage can increase the stretchiness of your perineal tissues and prepare you for the sensations of crowning during the birth. The massage can be done daily in the last weeks of pregnancy, by oiling your thumbs and placing them in your vagina. Breathe in, and as you breathe out press gently, using your thumb as a lever and encouraging the perineum to stretch.

- Touch your baby as it comes out to help you accept what is happening to your body.

- Take your time. There is no need to hurry – place trust in the natural process.

- You can wear as much or as little as you wish. You may get cold feet so put some socks on.

WHAT DAD MIGHT FEEL AND CAN DO

- Encourage her to stay upright. This will open up her pelvis, speed the birth, and reduce the risk of the baby becoming distressed.

- Encourage her to push only when she needs to and don't tell her to do it.

- Try making deep long "ahhh" sounds with her.

- If there is a pause between the first stage of labour and the birth, encourage her to rest. This lull may last minutes or longer, and providing there is no distress to mother or baby, it is advisable to wait.

- Keep her energy levels high with sugary drinks or tea with honey.

- Try dabbing her head with a wet cloth or give her a sponge to suck.

- Keep the room dark. She will be able to relax deeper if she feels less "on view". Keep the room quiet so that she can turn inward.

- Try to resist pressures from staff who might want her to lie flat on the bed unless there is an urgent medical need. If she is tired, she can give birth on her side with you supporting her legs.

- Try using supporting words and phrases from your preparations together.

- Encourage her to keep her jaw relaxed, lips soft, and face free from tension.

- Remain supportive, flexible, and positive. Soon you will be welcoming your baby.

Positions for giving birth

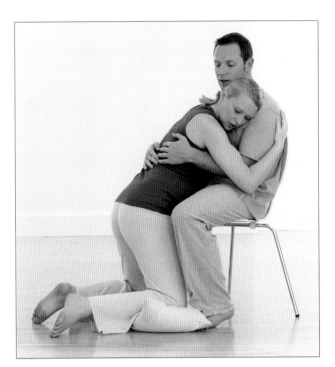

◄ Kneeling forward with head in partner's lap

You may like to birth your baby in the arms of your partner. This provides an upright position, which makes use of the benefits of gravity, and allows you to have your partner's support. You will feel safe in this position, while your partner holds you and breathes with you. You can come further upright if you need more gravity to assist with the birth.

While your partner sits in a chair, lean forward from your knees into his arms. Make sure you have cushions under your knees and one under your chest if you need it. You can take one leg up into **half kneeling, half squatting** (see below) if this helps make more space.

Half kneeling, half squatting ► (leaning onto a bean bag)

This is an open position close to the ground. You can happily labour while leaning into a bean bag or on your hands and knees. Have plenty of padding under your knees such as a yoga mat and cushions. Your midwife can see everything that she needs to and you are vertical, making the best use of gravity.

From an upright kneeling position, lift one knee up into a half kneeling, half squatting position. Gently lean forward onto a bean bag. As you focus on your breath rock backward and forward.

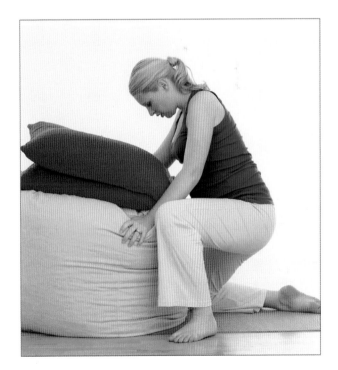

On all fours ▶

Birthing on your hands and knees is natural and is particularly helpful if the labour and birth are fast. You will have more control and your baby will descend a little more slowly.

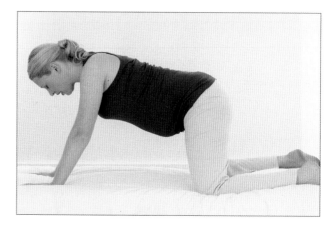

◀ **Kneeling on bed**

If you have been labouring on the bed, you can easily go up onto your knees while your partner stands at the side of the bed. Lean into him and hold him for support. This is a good upright birthing position.

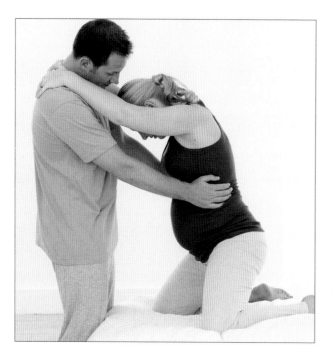

TIP Focus on gravity – if you imagine pushing down into the ground your pelvic floor will relax.

Lying on your side ▶

Giving birth while lying on your side is helpful if you are feeling exhausted. Make sure you have lots of cushions under your head and body and that your raised leg is supported by your birth partner. This position doesn't make the most of gravity, but it can slow down birthing if it is fast.

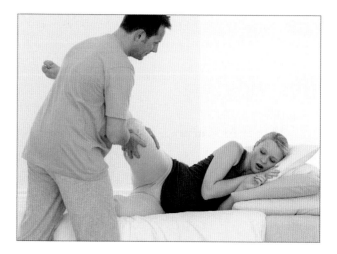

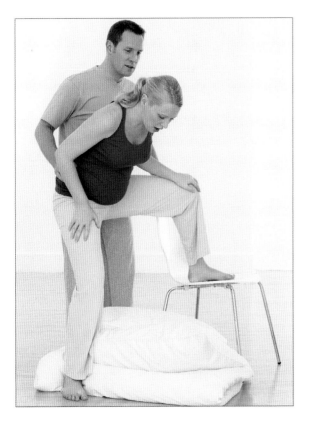

◄ Foot on chair

You may want to stand during birth. If you suffer from symphysis pubis dysfunction (see glossary) or if your baby is big, standing is a good way to speed up your birth.

Place the sole of one foot up on a chair, with your knee bent. Make sure the chair is steady and you have plenty of cushions and blankets on the floor. Some midwives may not be experienced or happy with this position, so check with them beforehand.

TIP For the supported squat, your partner shouldn't wear shoes, and he should also take off his socks to avoid slipping and injuring himself – and you.

Supported squat ►

The standing supported squat makes use of gravity and is the most effective position to encourage your baby's rapid descent.

1 Ask your partner to place his feet hip width apart.

2 Your partner should stand behind you, bend his knees, and lean back just a little so that your weight is carried against his pelvis.

3 Tell him to keep his back straight, and with his shoulders and arms relaxed, link your hands together under your arms, with his palms facing up.

4 Hold onto him. Focus on long, slow breaths and try the "ahhh" sounds as your baby starts to be birthed.

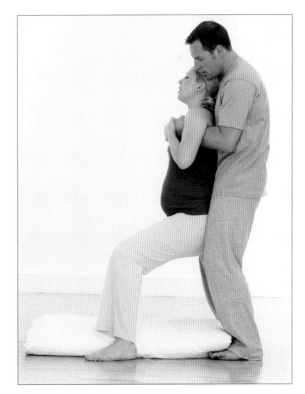

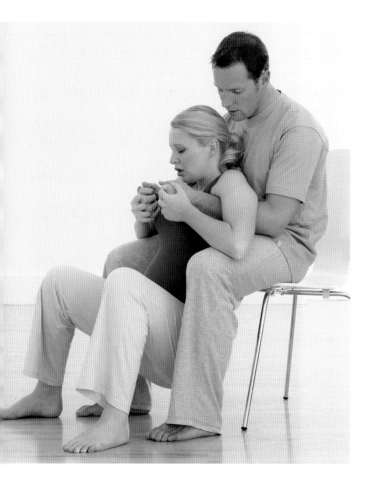

◄ Squat on a chair

This squat is useful if your partner has back problems and needs support. It is an easy, comfortable position.

1 Squat between your partner's knees, using his body for support. Your partner should sit forward onto the edge of the chair with knees wide open.

2 Your partner should keep his shoulders and arms relaxed, and link your hands together under your arms, with his palms facing upward.

3 Hold onto him. Focus on long, slow breaths and try the "ahhh" sounds as your baby starts to be birthed.

Kneeling on the bed with support ► of partner and midwife

Using the support of two people for birthing can be helpful and allows you to be supported in an upright position, as well as emotionally looked after.

Kneel on the bed with your knees apart. Put one arm around your partner and the other around your midwife or other birth companion. They can sit on the sides of the bed or stand, whatever feels most comfortable.

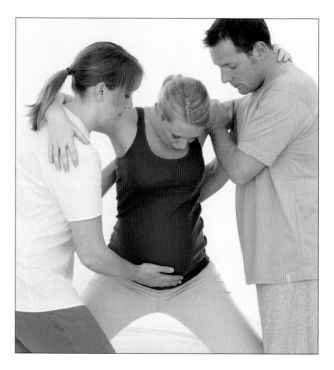

What if I'm in hospital?

In a hospital you can use these positions on the bed.

Use **kneeling on bed** (see page 66) and remember you can labour on your hands and knees.

The **supported squat** (see page 67) can speed up birth. **Kneeling on the bed with support of partner and midwife** (see page 68) can help both physically and emotionally.

Lying on your side (see page 66) is a valuable position if you are tired.

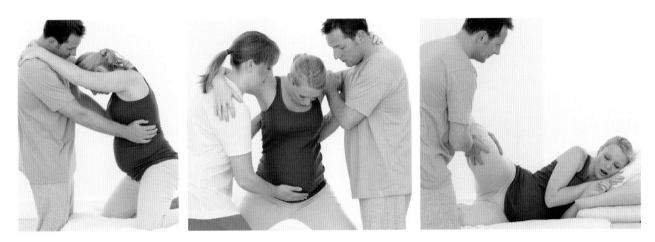

What if I'm at home?

At home you are free to use all the furniture and rooms to find the position to suit you.

Kneeling forwards with head in partner's lap position (see page 65) is intimate. You can take the chair into whichever room you wish.

If you were labouring on your hands and knees, get up into **half kneeling, half squatting** (see page 65).

Women who birth with **foot on chair** (see page 67) are aided by lots of use of gravity, so make sure there is good padding, such as a duvet, on the floor.

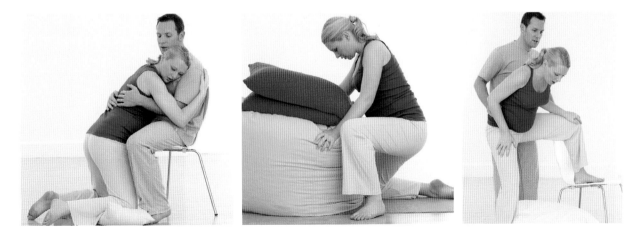

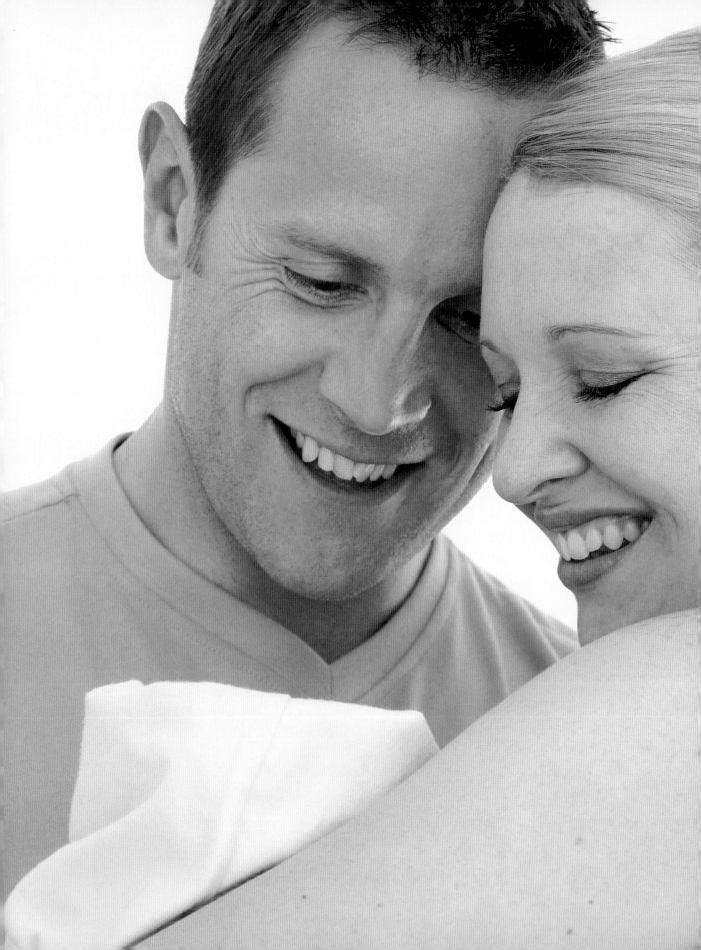

The third stage

That splendour of light which comes from the sun

Bhagavad Gita, Chapter 15, Verse 12

The third stage of labour

Your baby has been born. In these amazing moments you will be touching, cuddling, and discovering your baby for the first time. These first few moments are vital to the attachment process that takes place between you, so don't feel rushed and take your time. However, the birth of your baby does not mark the end of the birth – the placenta must still be birthed during the third stage of labour.

The best approach to a safe delivery of the placenta is a matter of debate. There is no absolute agreement on whether it is best to let it happen naturally unless there is excessive bleeding or to "actively manage" the third stage of pregnancy. A natural third stage of labour is one in which hormones are produced to birth the placenta. This happens most easily in a quiet, relaxed atmosphere. There you can hold your newborn baby in your arms and even breast-feed for the first time.

The chance of a natural third stage is greater if the rest of the labour and birth has so far taken place without intervention. You will probably birth your placenta in a similar position to that in which you gave birth to your baby, and using an upright position will encourage the placenta to be expelled – you can be supported to sit, squat, or kneel upright. You may

want to cuddle your baby at the same time – if this is the case, sitting up is more helpful. However, if you want to encourage the placenta to be expelled, you will need to be more upright, either standing or squatting. In this case your partner can hold the baby. The umbilical cord can remain attached to your baby until it has stopped pulsing, which will bring him or her the benefit of extra oxygenated blood.

Many hospitals prefer active management of the third stage of labour and may routinely inject the mother with oxytocin as the baby's first shoulder is being born. The drug acts to speed up the separation and expulsion of the placenta. Its routine use is said to have resulted in a dramatic drop in the incidence of post-partum haemorrhage (*see* glossary), which has been a serious cause of maternal illness, both in the past and in many developing countries today. Other people argue that the improvement might be due to better housing, sanitation, and general health. Also women are tending to have fewer babies – and risks are known to be less when this is the case.

REASONS FOR ACTIVE MANAGEMENT

Although you may want to deliver your placenta naturally, there are situations in which this is not possible. It may be advisable to opt for active management of the third stage of labour if you have:

- a multiple pregnancy (where you are pregnant with twins or triplets)
- had four or more previous babies
- too much amniotic fluid (polyhydramnios)

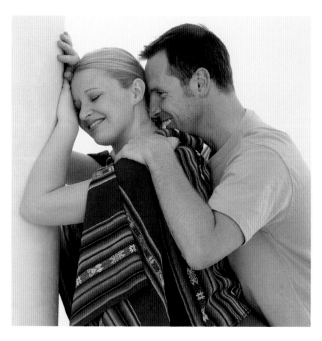

LEFT Once you have birthed the placenta, all the stages of labour are completed. Well done – you've done it!

- antepartum haemorrhage (bleeding after the 24th week of pregnancy)
- anaemia or malnutrition
- uterine fibroids
- blood-clotting disorders
- a history of post-partum haemorrhage

In addition, certain situations that can occur during labour can interfere with the release of hormones or the natural functioning of the uterus. This might make a natural delivery of the placenta less appropriate. These might include:

- the use of syntocin to induce or speed up labour
- the use of an epidural or spinal anaesthesia
- assisted delivery with forceps or ventouse
- the use of pethidine or other narcotic drugs during delivery
- mild ineffective contractions during the second stage of labour
- having clamped or cut the baby's umbilical cord early
- if labour has been long

Time is of the essence when the third stage of labour is actively managed. When syntometrine (*see glossary*) is given it acts on the uterus, putting it into spasm and closing the cervix in 4 to 7 minutes. The midwife will therefore be in a hurry to ensure the placenta is delivered within the time available before the cervix closes. Other measures are taken during active management, such as immediate clamping and cutting of the cord, to prevent the baby from being over-perfused with blood, and controlled cord traction (pulling) to help the expulsion of the placenta.

One thing which is not disputed is that natural and active management methods should not be mixed. In the natural process the midwife should "sit on her hands" and avoid intervening. Feel free to discuss these issues beforehand with your midwife.

WHAT'S GOING ON?

As your baby is born, your levels of oxytocin will peak, but they won't diminish immediately. Stimulated by suckling your baby, strong contractions will continue, reducing the volume of the uterus, and the placenta will separate from the rapidly shrinking uterine wall.

Once the placenta is detached, the contractions continue until the placenta is pushed out. There is likely to be a certain amount of bleeding from the site where the placenta had embedded itself, but the contracting muscle fibres of the uterus will shut down the blood vessels. The body also produces high levels of coagulants to clot the blood and protect you from haemorrhage. An hour afterward, your uterus will have been reduced to the size of a grapefruit. By the time of your six-week postnatal check, it will be back to its normal size. If the third stage of labour is actively managed, an injection of syntometrine will put the uterus into spasm so that the placenta is delivered quickly.

BREATHING TIPS FOR THE THIRD STAGE

Women describe birthing the placenta in different ways – some feel the contractions are painful, while others say it doesn't hurt at all or even find the experience pleasurable. The placenta is about one-third of the weight of your baby and easier to deliver. You may be so "wrapped up" with cuddling your baby that you won't need to focus on your breathing. But if you need to, try a long, slow in breath, touching and preferably feeding your baby, and release a long, slow out breath. Often the placenta will come out with just one or two gentle out breaths.

Helpful hints for the third stage

WHAT MUM MIGHT FEEL AND CAN DO

- Congratulations – your baby is here! Take your time to enjoy your baby's presence because these first few moments are vital to bonding. Feel free to be a tigress and defend your territory – all non-emergency checks can wait.

- Try to place your bare baby close to you for skin-to-skin contact and offer breast milk to help the expulsion of the placenta. Don't worry if your baby isn't interested in feeding straight away – you can try again a little later.

- Remember that it's normal to feel a mixture of emotions. Be kind to yourself. It can take a while for everything to sink in.

- You may want to kneel or go into any upright position for the birth of the placenta.

- If you have a sore perineum, try calendula tincture. Homeopathy can also be helpful, especially for aches. Consult a homeopath for more advice.

- Breast-feeding is the best way to continue the close relationship with your baby that you have formed in pregnancy, and breast milk is the best food for your baby. It's normal to find breast-feeding difficult so be persistent about asking your midwife for help. Breast-feeding takes practice.

- It's usual to have afterbirth pains when you breast-feed, especially if you've had more than one child. This is because the release of oxytocin will cause your uterus to contract. Within a few days it will get better. If it's really bad, try your long, slow breath practice whenever you feel pain.

WHAT DAD MIGHT FEEL AND CAN DO

- Congratulations – your baby is here! You may be feeling a mixture of emotions – excitement and joy, as well as apprehension and uncertainty, but this is to be expected. Be kind to yourself.

- Your partner needs to be allowed to inspect her baby in the most private way. This means keeping noise levels down and "lying low". You may want to ask the midwives for some privacy. Routine checks can wait unless there is an emergency.

- Encourage your partner to be in an upright position while the placenta is delivered. You may want to cut the cord. This can be an emotional action: it symbolizes your baby's independence and confirms your role as a parent.

- Your partner may feel shivery after the birth. Keep her warm. An overhead heater can be useful.

- Feel free to have skin to skin contact with your baby. This will encourage you and your baby to get to know each other.

- Be understanding of your partner's moods. In the early days, she may have a mixture of emotions that swing up and down. Her body has been through a tremendous amount in the last few days.

- Get some rest yourself. You will feel tired if you have supported her throughout the labour and birth. Enjoy these precious moments as a family – they will pass quickly.

Positions in the third stage of labour

Kneeling on floor ▸

If you had your baby on the floor in a kneeling position, you will most likely want to stay on the floor to cuddle him or her. If this is the case, you can kneel as you breast-feed your baby and then get up onto your knees when you feel ready to birth the placenta.

TIP Your birth partner can help you in the third stage by making sure the environment around you is quiet, warm, and dimly lit.

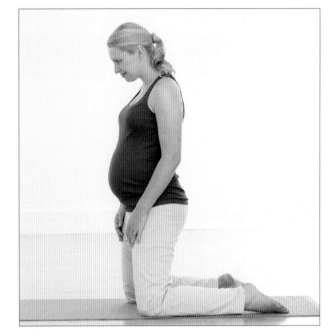

◂ Squatting

You may want to squat if you used squatting during the birth.

You can squat unaided over a dish. With a gentle push the placenta will come out. You may need help in the squatting positions – your partner can cuddle the baby and your midwife can assist you.

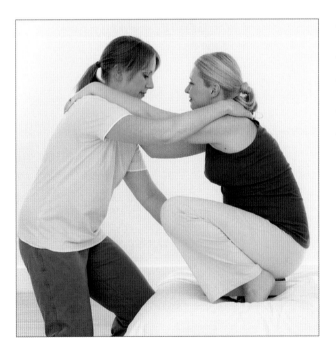

Leaning into bed ▶

If you are on the bed, you may want to lean into it. Your partner can help you by making sure you are upright and comfortable.

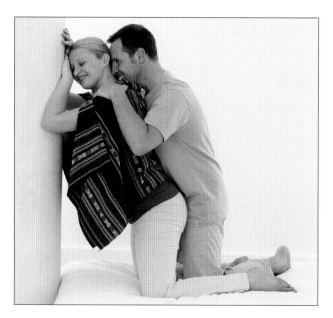

TIP You may feel shivery or cold, so make sure your partner has a blanket ready to wrap around you.

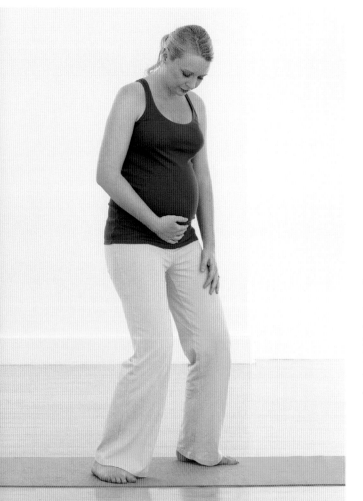

◀ Standing

If you have had your baby standing up, you may want to get up when you feel the urge to birth the placenta. If this is the case, try **supported squats** (*see* page 67) with the help of your partner, or just standing with your legs slightly bent. Once the placenta is out you will want to relax and lie down on your side with your baby beside you.

Sitting upright

This position helps the placenta to separate and the fluids to drain from the uterus. You can cuddle and feed your baby in this position. If you are in bed, you may want to use this position to deliver the placenta. If you lift up your leg and turn onto your side or come up to one of the more upright positions, it will help the delivery of the placenta.

Putting it all together

The following pages show how you can choose a sequence for labour and birth, depending on whether you are at home or in hospital. They are meant only as a guide, so you can adapt them to suit your needs.

HOME BIRTH

Walking can speed up the first stage, or you may want to lean into a wall or use the sofa, with your partner massaging you. Some women prefer to be on their hands and knees. When you need to bear down, you can push on a bean bag. A half kneeling, half squat position uses gravity to help birth your baby.

First stage of labour
Walking (see page 43)

Leaning into a wall (see page 44)
Upright kneeling position on a sofa (see page 56)

Transition stage of labour
On all fours (see page 47)
Resting forward on a bean bag (see page 47)

Birth of your baby
Half kneeling, half squatting (see page 65)

Suggestions for a home birth

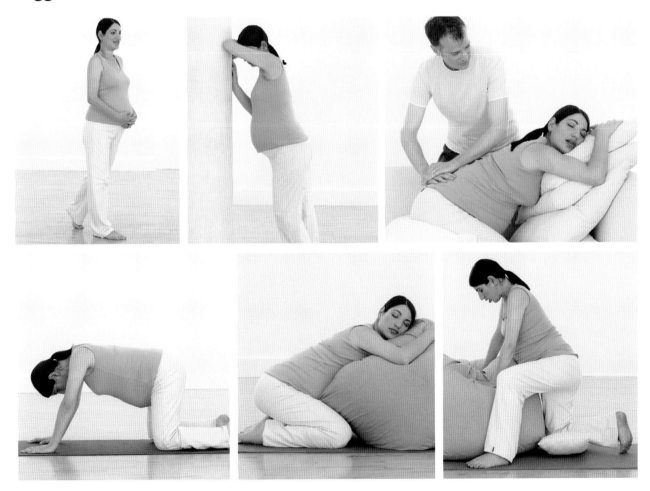

Suggestions for a birth in a hospital or a birthing unit

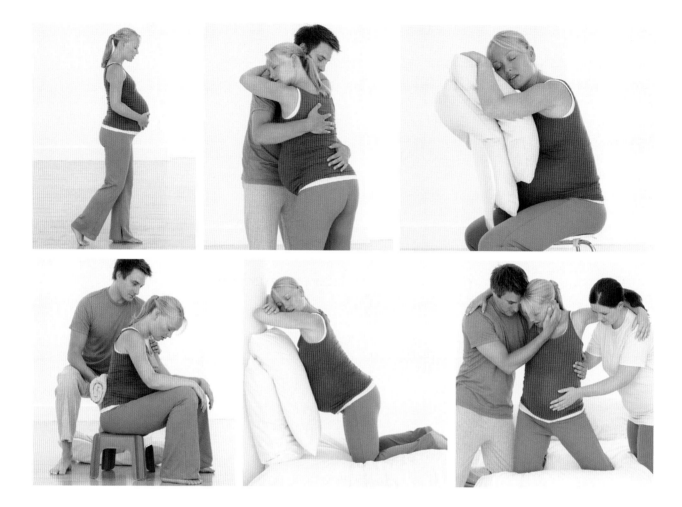

BIRTH IN HOSPITAL OR A BIRTHING UNIT

Try to walk a little bit to quicken your labour, resting between contractions in the arms of your partner. As labour becomes more intense, try resting forward on a chair. Try using water to help you relax, even in a hospital. Your partner could come in with you. As labour intensifies, rest forward onto the bed head. You may want to be massaged or left alone. With the support of your birth partners, you can birth in a supported kneeling position to make use of gravity. It can also be used for birthing the placenta.

First stage of labour
Walking (see page 43)
Couple's embrace (see page 46)
Sitting astride a chair (see page 45)

Transition stage of labour
Shower on a stool or chair (see page 49)
Upright kneeling position (see page 56)

Birth of your baby
Kneeling with support of partner and midwife (see page 68)

HOSPITAL BIRTH WHEN TIRED OR ANXIOUS

If your labour is slow, try walking to speed it up. You can go outside for fresh air, or at least walk around the ward. For labour to pick up, you may need to be left in peace. Dim the lights, close the door, and turn to your breath. As labour progresses and you become more tired, you may want to use a chair. Your partner can massage you and apply hot, wet towels to your back. Between contractions, rest by leaning forward – this helps to slow labour down if it feels fast. If you feel too tired to continue, lie on your side – not on your back. You can give birth to your baby lying on your side if your partner supports your top leg.

First stage of labour
Walking (see page 43)
Use the toilet for privacy (see page 48)
Using a chair and a bed for support (see page 45)

Transition stage of labour
Upright kneeling position (see page 56)
Leaning forward onto the bed (see page 58)

Birth of your baby
Lying on your side (see page 66)

Suggestions for a hospital birth when tired or anxious

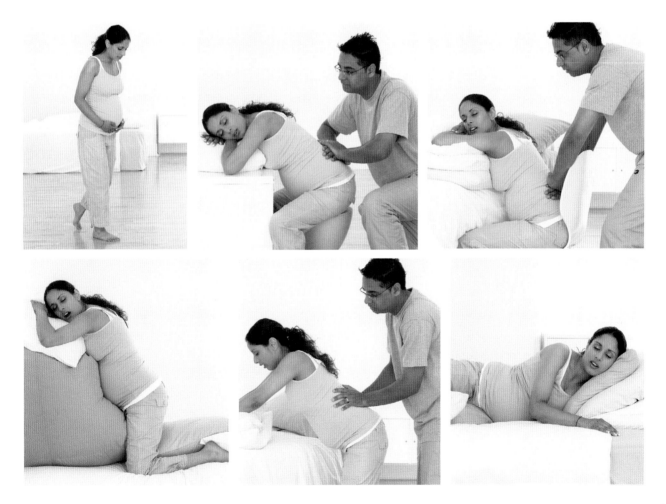

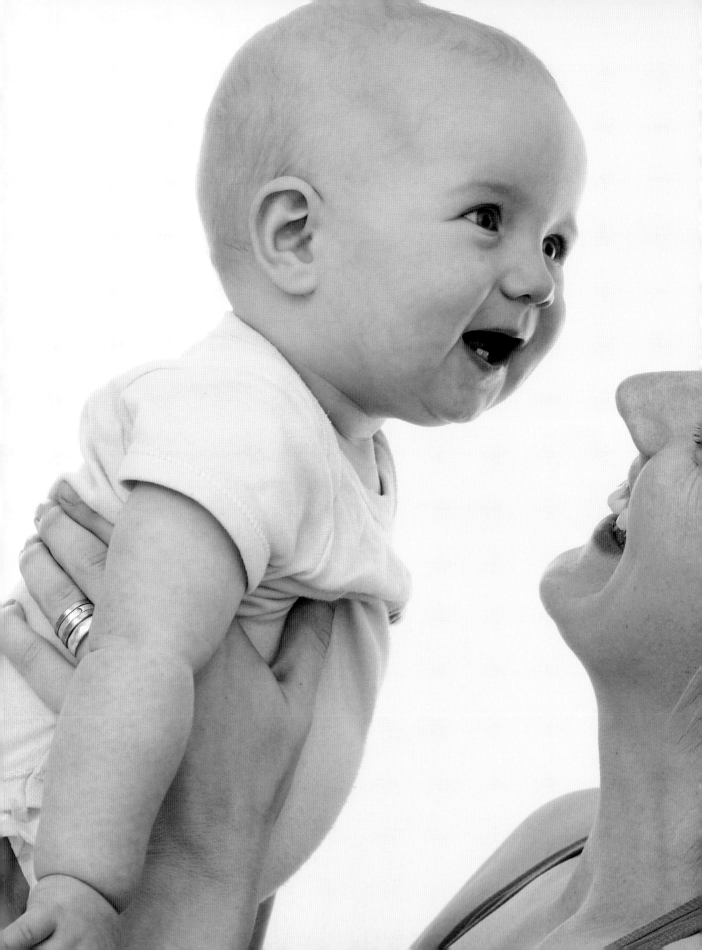

What now?

With light, above, below, across, so shines
The Lord of Love and fills the hearts
of all created beings

Shvetashvatara Upanishad, Chapter 5, Verse 4

What now?

Congratulations! Your birth is complete and your baby is now here. As a new mother you will likely be overwhelmed, and you will be amazed at how this beautiful baby can turn your life upside down. Yoga also has a role to play after the birth in providing harmony and balance – which is exactly what a woman needs after she has had her baby.

Whatever birth you have experienced, yoga can continue to provide benefits to you and your baby. Yoga can help you to reconnect with yourself. You will feel more refreshed, flexible and toned, and re-energized. Yoga can help you to get back into shape in a gentle way that respects your body.

The physical benefits will be an improved posture, stronger lower back, pelvic floor (which can be especially important if you are suffering from stress incontinence), and abdominal muscles, which may feel under strain from feeding and carrying your baby. Gentle stretches can relieve tension from your shoulders and neck, and will give you a poise and grace that will help you to embrace motherhood. The emotional benefits are huge. Your hormones will be fluctuating, and with the joy of motherhood there may also come the lack of sleep, difficulties with breast-feeding, and a sense of loss of freedom. All of these feelings are normal as long as they are not excessive. If you feel persistently down, you should seek help.

Your practice of yoga can help you to find a way to recuperate and refresh yourself, especially through joined relaxation with your baby. The breathing used in pregnancy can also help you stay focused and calm, providing a pause from hectic life and helping you remain centred. Doing yoga with your baby will improve your communication, enabling you to interact with him or her in a way that your baby will love. In time, your baby will be able to imitate you when you are on your yoga mat being a cat or a dog. The fun you have will be mutual and you will both look forward to your yoga practice together. You will be able to connect at a deep, profound level, and this shared understanding will grow.

Before you do this practice, be sure of the following:

- Make sure that you and your baby have been for your six-week post-natal check up.
- If you have had a Caesarean, go slowly. You should leave out the **alternate leg raises** (see page 86) and **mini bridge** (see page 87) and focus on **reverse breathing** (see page 88) and pelvic floor exercises.
- If you do practice with your baby, be open to his or her moods and stop if your baby cries. Don't give up completely – try again later.
- Create your own lovely secure space. This could be the same as in pregnancy. Unroll your yoga mat, turn off the phone, and focus on your baby and your practice.
- Remember it's better to do little yoga sessions often rather than a long one only once in a while.
- Be gentle and patient with yourself. Respect your body, and with time your strength will return.
- Have fun and enjoy the sessions with your baby. Woof like a dog! Meow like a cat! Lie down like a pancake!

TIP Don't struggle alone if you feel low after having a baby. Many women "have the blues" at this time and networking with others may help you. Don't be afraid to seek professional medical help if necessary.

Movements and positions for mother and baby

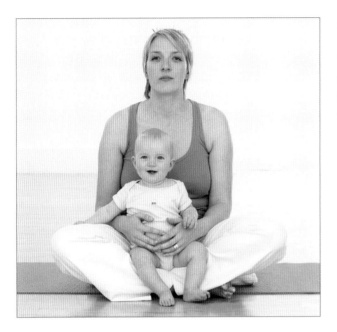

◄ **Centring for you with your baby**

This focuses on stabilizing the emotions and calming the mind before beginning your yoga. Don't worry if your baby distracts you – you will soon learn to centre yourself with him or her there.

1 With your baby in your arms or lying next to you on your mat, sit as upright as you can. If you are tense, take a deep in breath and as you breathe out, release a big "ha!" breath. Do this a few times.

2 Close your eyes and start to focus on each in breath and out breath. Gradually start to deepen your in breath and lengthen your out breath. Focus on this as long as you feel comfortable. Slowly bring your breath back to normal and open your eyes.

Lying down spinal twist ▼

This lovely twist can tone the spine and strengthen the legs. It can also be relaxing.

1 Begin by lying down with your knees bent, your head to the centre, and your baby lying on the mat next to you. Straighten your arms, with your palms facing upward. Take a breath in.

2 As you breathe out, gently drop your knees to your right and turn your head to your left. Relax. Bring your knees and head back to centre as you breathe in.

3 On your next out breath, drop your knees to the other side. Repeat a few times.

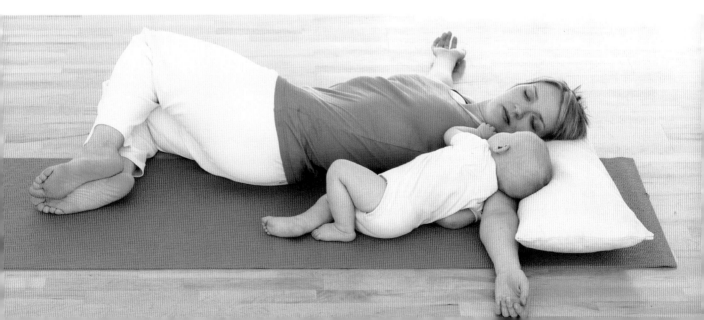

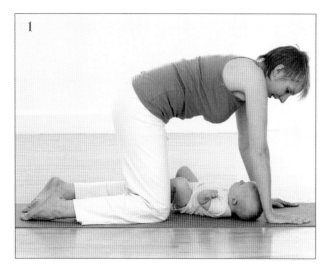

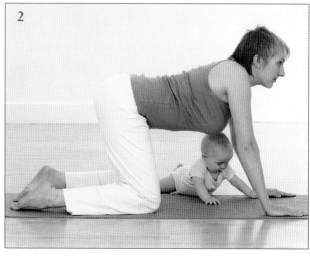

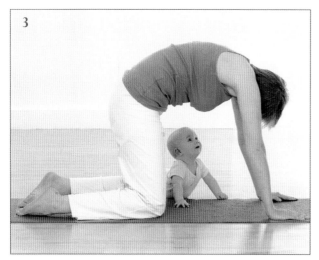

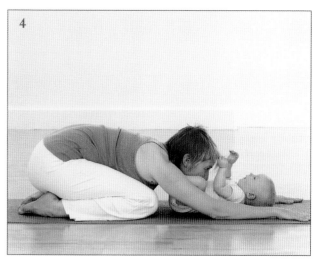

Cat with baby ▲

Here is a chance to stretch your back, warm your body, and stimulate circulation.

1 Begin on all fours, with your shoulders over your wrists and your hips over your knees. Keep your weight evenly distributed between your hands and knees. Draw your tummy in toward your spine. Spread your fingers apart and press into the floor.

2 As you inhale slowly arch your back, bringing your tail bone and head up toward the ceiling.

3 As you exhale slowly reverse the posture, rounding your back and tucking your tail bone and chin in toward your body. Repeat three or four times.

4 When you finish rest in the extended child pose, with your bottom on your heels and your arms stretched in front of you.

TIP For both of these positions, your baby can lie on the mat directly below your chest, so you can make eye contact.

▼ Downward dog with baby

1 Start in the **cat with baby** (see opposite) neutral position, neither arched nor rounded. With your fingers spread wide, distribute your weight evenly through your hands and knees.

2 Spread your feet apart almost to the width of the yoga mat. Tuck your toes under and lift your hips toward the ceiling. Straighten your legs, move your thighs back, and lift your knees. Reach down and back with your heels and stretch your toes forward.

Draw your tummy in toward your spine. Allow your neck and head to relax, letting it drop toward your baby. You can say a "hello" to your baby and make dog sounds.

3 When you've had enough, slowly bend your knees so you are back on your hands and knees. Bring your bottom to your heels and rest in the extended child pose with your arms stretched out in front of you, for as long as you feel comfortable.

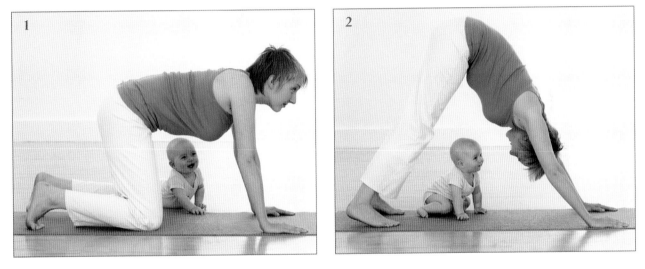

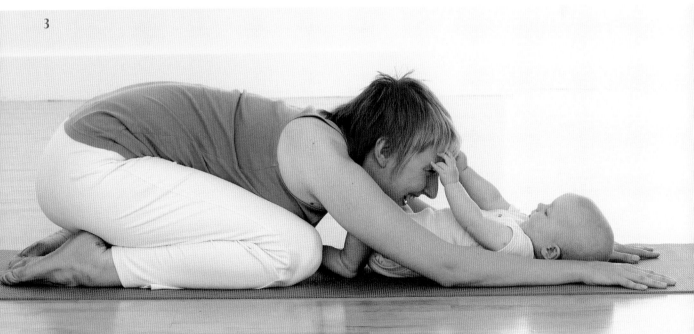

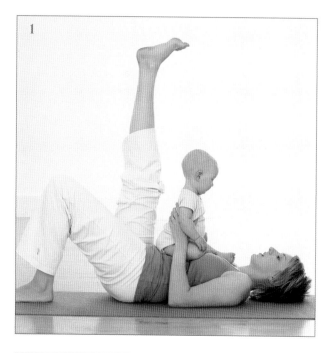

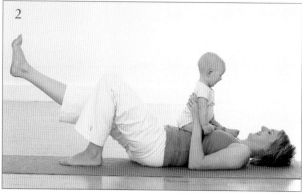

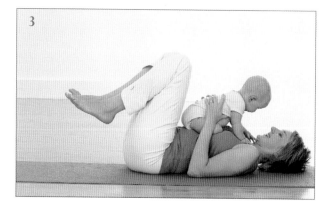

◄ Alternate leg raises

This is a gentle pose to do with your baby. It will strengthen your abdominal muscles. Go gently and stop if there is any pain.

1 Lie on your mat with your legs bent. Your baby can sit or lie on your chest as you support him or her. Draw your tummy in toward your spine as you breathe in. Straighten your right leg and lift it toward the ceiling.

2 As you breathe out, slowly lower your right leg back down to the ground. Bring your knee toward your chest and begin again. Repeat this a few times and then change to the other leg.

3 When you finish, bring both knees toward you and gently rock from side to side, using the motion to massage your back. Remember to continue to support your baby.

TIP If you want to strengthen your deep abdominal muscles and tone your pelvic floor – both of which were under strain during your pregnancy and your baby's birth – these two exercises are essential.

▼ Mini bridge

1 Lie on your back with your knees bent and feet on the floor close to your bottom. Place your baby sitting on your tummy, supported with your hands under his or her armpits.

2 Breathe in and press your feet into the ground. Lift your hips and roll up slowly through your spine, moving your hip bones toward the ceiling. Stay here for a moment and when you're ready roll back slowly, trying to feel each vertebra as it makes contact with the mat. Repeat a few times.

3 Bring your knees toward you and gently rock from side to to side when you're finished, using the motion to massage your back.

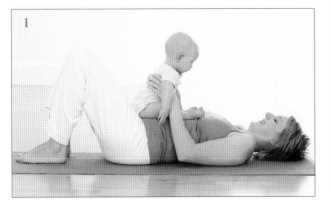

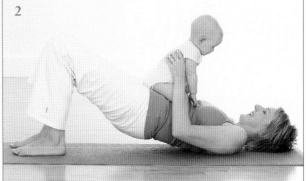

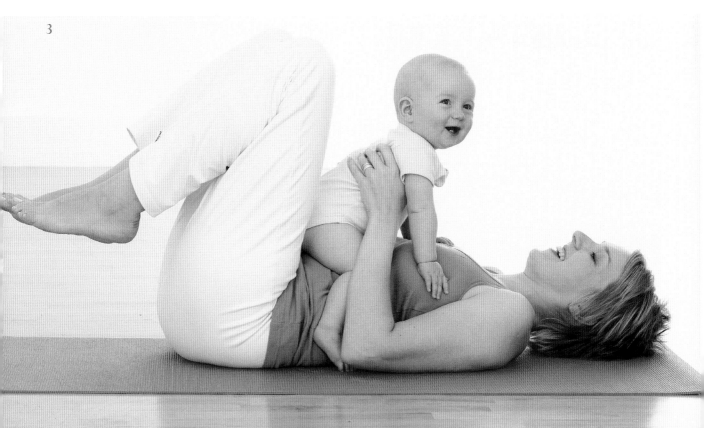

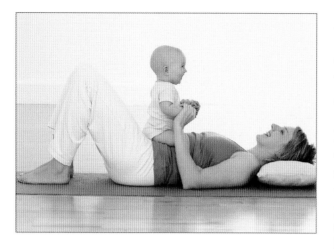

◄ Reverse breathing

This breathing practice can be used straight after the birth (even if you have had a Caesarean section) and is a good way to gently tone deep abdominal muscles.

Lie on your back with your knees bent and put a cushion under your neck if you need it. Lie your baby across your tummy, or support him or her against your thighs. Breathe in deeply. As you breathe out, draw your tummy muscles inward, toward the base of your spine. Repeat this a few times and stop when you've had enough.

Relaxing together ▼

Regularly practising joined relaxation with your baby can be important to help stop tensions accumulating. This is essential if you are a working mum or have other children, because there is seldom much time to recharge your batteries and enjoy being with your baby. Try this with your baby and ideally as a family.

1 Lie on your back. You can place a pillow under your head and bend your knees to protect your back. Rest your baby across your chest or lie him or her next to you. Your partner and/or other children may want to lie alongside you. Take a few moments to release any tension by breathing in deeply and as you breathe out making "ha!" sounds.

2 Begin to focus on each in breath and out breath. Allow your breathing to soften and your body to release tension. Your baby may make noises – this is normal. If she cries, stop and comfort her and try again later. When you finish, have a gentle stretch.

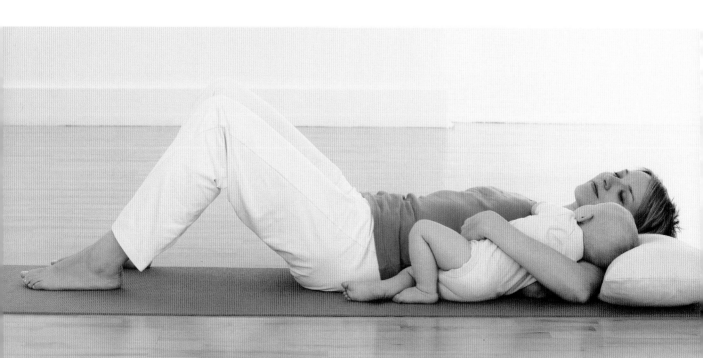

Testimonials

"Yoga breathing techniques helped me to remain calm and positive throughout my labour."

Yasia Williams

"When I found out that I was pregnant I decided to take up yoga. Practising yoga each week helped me to stay supple and flexible, and also helped me to have a a positive outlook and approach to childbirth. When I went into labour, yoga helped me keep focused and relaxed." *Lucy Webb*

"Thanks to Julie I had an oasis of time each week in which to prepare physically and mentally for the greatest physical challenge of my life. Yoga gave me confidence in the face of the unknown." *Cathy Mattis*

"During yoga classes with Julie I learnt the positions that can help labour to progress naturally, and how breathing helps with pain and anxiety. When I went into labour I felt liberated. By focusing on my breathing I was able to remain calm and in control." *Cath Calvert*

"From a father's perspective I have found that yoga techniques gave me a focus, so that I could be more actively involved, and I felt more confident with my role during the labour." *Nick Calvert*

"I have no doubt that yoga helped me to prepare mentally and physically for labour and the birth. I felt in control." *Sameena Ayub*

Glossary

Adrenaline   A hormone released by the adrenal glands in response to stress. It increases the pulse and respiration, and prepares the body for physical action.

Anaemia   An abnormally low amount of red blood cells, leading to reduced oxygen supply to the body and tiredness.

Asana   A body pose or posture used in yoga. It forms the suffix in the names of various yoga poses, for example *Tadasana* (the mountain pose) and *Shavasana*.

Bhagavad Gita   A key ancient Hindu scripture, meaning the "lord's song". It contains teachings on the meaning of yoga.

Braxton-Hicks contractions   Normal painless and periodic tightenings of the muscles of the uterus, which occur in at random intervals from the middle of pregnancy, in preparation for labour.

Caesarean birth   Either a planned or emergency surgical procedure which can be used when a vaginal birth is not advised. A cut about 20cm (8in) long is made in the lower abdomen and the womb is opened to release the baby.

Doula   A paid assistant who attends the labour, and can provide the mother with physical and emotional assistance before, during, or after the birth.

Endorphins   Natural brain chemicals which produce a state of improved mood and reduced pain, especially after exercise and deep breathing.

Episiotomy   The practice of cutting the perineum during hospital delivery, the intention being to enlarge the outlet and prevent tears. However the procedure has shown to be a risk factor for tears, incontinence and delayed healing.

Fibroid   Muscle cells or other tissues that grow slowly within the wall of the uterus. They can be symptom free but can also cause bleeding, discomfort, and reproductive problems.

Hatha yoga   A popular type of yoga that uses breathing practices, or *pranayama*, and a wide range of body postures. Ha-tha means "sun"-"moon" – a fusion of opposites.

Intervention   Artificial assistance by a medical procedure when natural processes such as birth are not going well or not going to plan.

Lithotomy position   The position of lying flat on the back with the knees bent and held in position raised above the hips, with the thighs apart. The position was popular with obstetricians for birthing in times gone by but is restrictive for women and is no longer recommended.

Namaste   A gesture made by bringing together the palms of both hands before the heart with fingers pointing up and head slightly bowed. Derived from the Sanskrit words "nama" meaning "bend" and "te" meaning "you", it is used as a humble and straightforward greeting.

Occipito-anterior position   The back of your baby's head is facing the front of your pelvis as it comes down the birth canal. This is the easiest position for delivery.

Occipito-posterior position   The back of your baby's head is facing the rear of your pelvis as it comes down the birth canal. This delivery position can be slower and cause more back ache in labour.

Om   A chant consisting of three sounds, "a", "u" and "m". A sacred sound in ancient Indian religion, one which drives away cluttered thoughts, brings relaxation and renews energy. The "om" represents the everything from which the universe was made.

Oxytocin   A hormone which strengthens uterine contractions in labour and stimulates breast milk production during suckling. Its release is easiest in stress-free environments and is promoted by vaginal and nipple stimulation.

Pelvic floor   A group of muscles in the base of the pelvis, important in childbirth, sexual function, urination and defecation. The pelvic floor is a sling of muscles, stretching from the pubic bone to the tail bone, which supports the pelvic contents and has openings for the bladder, bowel and womb.

Perineum   The area of skin between the vagina and the anus.

Pethidine   A drug used to provide pain relief, given by injection into the thigh or buttock.

Postnatal depression   Unlike the "baby blues", which are mild and very common in the few days after giving birth, postnatal depression is longer-lasting, deeper, and may need professional treatment. In the "baby blues" many women experience mood swings, crying, irritability, restlessness, and lowness. In postnatal depression there may be stronger feelings of anxiety, despair, anger, and sadness that can last for months. There may also be changes in weight, inability to concentrate, feelings of worthlessness, and a loss of interest in normal daily life.

Prana   An ancient Hindu term referring to life force energy which is found in all aspects of nature. It is the vital air or breath of the human body as well as the life force of the universe.

Pranayama   Breathing techniques used in yoga to calm the mind and strengthen the prana (life energy).

Preeclampsia   High maternal blood pressure, occurring during pregnancy, anytime after the 16th week but especially close to the birth. Most cases are mild but there can be risks for mother and baby.

Reverse breathing   A breathing practice that helps to restore deep muscle tone and that is especially helpful after Caesarean birth. Breath is inhaled in the normal way and as it is exhaled the navel is drawn toward the spine.

Stress incontinence   A leakage of urine when there is extra pressure (or stress) on the bladder. Most commonly it is due to weakened pelvic floor muscles, especially after pregnancy. The leakage is most obvious during coughing, laughing or exercise.

Symphysis pubis   A cartilage joint between the left and right sides of the bony pelvis, easily felt at the front of the body, just below the bladder. It stretches open slightly during birth.

Symphysis pubis dysfunction   When the ligaments in the symphysis pubis loosen too much before birth, leading to instability in the pelvic joints. This can be made worse as the baby grows and increases in weight, and results in mild to severe pain.

Syntocin   A synthetic form of the hormone oxytocin, used to artificially induce labour.

Syntometrine   A drug which is used to manage the third stage of labour, promoting strong uterine contractions to birth the placenta.

Ventouse   A vacuum device used to help the delivery of a your baby when assistance is needed.

List of useful organizations

Antenatal Results and Choices (ARC)
73 Charlotte Street,
London, W1T 4PN
Tel: 020 7631 0280
www.arc-uk.org
Provides support and information to parents throughout the antenatal testing process.

Birth and Bonding International (Doula association)
60 Nottingham Road,
Belper, DE56 1JH
Tel: 01773 826055
Has a list of doulas, who are paid birth supporters.

Birthlight
PO Box 148,
Cambridge, CB4 2GB
Tel: 01223 362288
www.birthlight.com
Provides a network of trained teachers in antenatal, post-natal and baby yoga.

British Homeopathic Association
Hehnemann House, 29 Park Street
West, Luton, LU1 3BE
Tel: 0870 4443950
www.trusthomeopathy.org
Information and a list of practitioners.

British Wheel of Yoga
25 Jermyn Street,
Sleaford, NG34 7RU
Tel: 01592 306851
www.bwy.org.uk
Provides a list of yoga teachers in the UK.

Caesarean Support Network
55 Cooil Drive, Douglas,
Isle of Man, IM2 2HF
Tel: 01624 661269
www.ukselfhelp.info/caesarean
Advice to mothers who have had or may need a Caesarean delivery.

Gingerbread
307 Borough High Street
London, SE1 1JH
Tel: 020 7403 9500
www.gingerbread.org.uk
Offers information, advice and support to single parents through a network of local groups.

Independent Midwives Association
89 Green Lane,
Farncombe, GU7 3TB
Tel: 01483 425833
www.independentmidwives.org.uk
Lobbies for the traditional role of the midwife and provides a list of midwives who will support home births.

La Leche League (Great Britain)
PO Box 29, West Bridgford,
Nottingham, NG2 7NP
Tel: 0845 456 1855
www.laleche.org.uk
Supports mothers with breastfeeding challenges.

Miscarriage Association
c/o Clayton Hospital, Northgate,
Wakefield, WF1 3JS
Tel: 01924 200799
www.miscarriageassociation.org.uk
Offers support and advice.

National Childbirth Trust (NCT)
Alexandra House, Oldham Terrace,
London, W3 6NH
Tel: 0870 770 3236
www.nctpregnancyandbabycare. com
Provides information and support.

One Parent Families
255 Kentish Town Road,
London, NW5 2LX
Tel: 0800 0185026
www.oneparentfamilies.org.uk
Information on financial, legal and housing problems.

Splashdown Water Birth Services Ltd
17 Wellington Terrace,
Harrow on the Hill, HA1 3EP
Tel: 08456 123405
www.waterbirth.co.uk
Provide pools for water births.

Vaginal Birth after Caesarean (VBAC)
8 Wren Way,
Farnborough, GU14 8SZ
Tel: 01243 868440
Information for women considering a vaginal birth after a Caesarean section.

Yoga Therapy Centre
90–92 Pentonville Road,
London, N1 9HS
Tel: 020 7689 3040
www.yogatherapy.org
The Yoga Biomedical Trust.

Bibliography

Balaskas, Janet, *New Active Birth: A Concise Guide to Natural Childbirth,* Harper Collins, London, 1990.

Balaskas, Janet, *Preparing for Birth with Yoga: Empowering and Effective Exercise for Pregnancy and Childbirth,* Thorsons, New York, 2003.

Balaskas, Janet, and Gordon, Yehudi, *The Encyclopaedia of Pregnancy and Birth,* Little, Brown and Co., London, 1989.

Farhi, Donna, *Yoga, Mind, Body and Spirit: a return to wholeness,* Henry Holt and Co., New York, 2000.

Freedman, Françoise, *Yoga for Pregnancy, Birth and Beyond,* Dorling Kindersley, London, 2004.

Freedman, Françoise and Hall, Doriel, *Yoga for Pregnancy and Mother's First Year,* Lorenz Books, Bath, 2003.

Gaskin, Ina, *Spiritual Midwifery,* Book Publishing Company, 2002.

Kitzinger, Sheila, *Rediscovering Birth,* Little, Brown and Co., London, 2000.

Kitzinger, Sheila, *Birth your Way: Choosing Birth at Home or in a Birth Centre,* Dorling Kindersley, London, 2002.

Leboyer, Frederick, *Birth without Violence,* Healing Arts Press, New York, 2002.

Llewellyn-Thomas, Julie, *Yoga for Mother and Baby,* Mitchell Beazley, London, 2006.

Priya, Jacqueline, *Birth Traditions and Modern Pregnancy Care,* Element Book Limited, Shaftsbury, 1992.

Robertson, Andrea, *The Midwife Companion: The art of support during birth,* ACE Graphics, Camperdown, 2002.

Saraswati, Swami, *Asana Pranayama Mudra Bandha,* Yoga Publications Trust, Munger Bulhar, India, 2002

Staton, Laura and Perron, Sarah, *Baby Om: Yoga for Mothers and Babies,* Henry Holt and Co., New York, 2002.

Teasdill, Wendy, *Yoga for Pregnancy,* Gaia, London, 2000.

Tew, Marjorie, *Safer Childbirth? A Critical History of Maternity Care,* Chapman and Hall, London, 1990.

Thomas, Pat, *Every Woman's Birth Rights,* Thorsons, London, 1996.

Wagner, Marsden, *Pursuing the Birth Machine,* ACE Graphics, 1994.

Wolf, Naomi, *Misconceptions, Truth, Lies and the Unexpected on the Journey to Motherhood,* Chatto and Windus, London, 2001.

World Health Organization, Department of Reproductive Health and Research, *Safe Motherhood, Care in Normal Birth: a practical guide,* WHO, Geneva.

Index

Author's acknowledgements

I would like to thank the team at Mitchell Beazley for all your hard work – especially Jon who put up with my endless phone calls. A huge thank you to Nicky who spent many hours making this book look as beautiful and special as it does (and for driving with huge bean bags stuffed into her car!)

Thank you to Ruth for your skill and patience, and Vicky for your great make-up work.

Thank you to Paul at Yogamatters who kindly lent us their beautiful clothes and yoga mats.

A very special thank you to all the models who patiently devoted their time and cheerfully breathed their way through many positions while we took the photos – without your generosity this book could not have happened.

On a more personal level, thank you to my teachers who have inspired my teachings. Françoise Freedman from Birthlight; Andre Wilson who helped me many years ago; Robin Monro from the Yoga Therapy Centre who enabled me to teach at the Royal Homeopathic Hospital; Great Ormond Street right at the very beginning; and Ralph, my teacher and inspiration.

Thank you to Giles who entertained our four children while I wrote! Most importantly, thank you to my four children, Clara, Rafi, Gabriel and Lucia – each one of your births have been precious and have laid the foundations for this book.